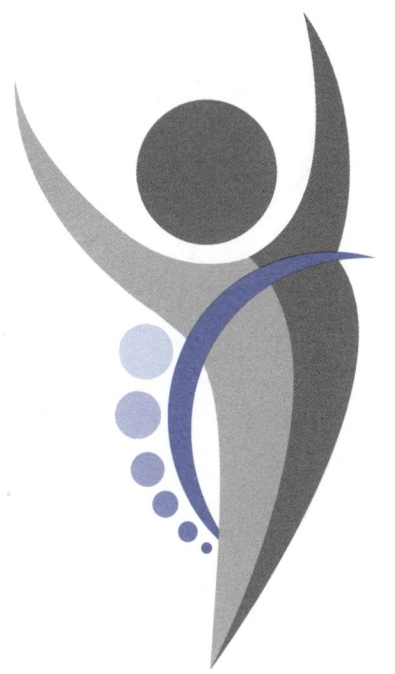

Power over Pain

Intelligent Fitness for the Amateur and Professional

by **Shereen D. Farber**
Ph.D., OTR, FAOTA, BFLT, WFLT

and **Debra S. Knapp**
CPT, ACE, AFAA, Certified Egoscue Posture,
Alignment & Pain Management Specialist

Published by:
Integrated Health Services-Indy

Distributed by:
Cardinal Publishers Group
2402 Shadeland Ave., Suite A
Indianapolis, IN 46219

in association with:
IBJ Book Publishing
41 E. Washington St., Suite 200
Indianapolis, IN 46204
www.ibjbp.com

Copyright 2014 by Shereen D. Farber, Ph.D., OTR, FAOTA, BFLT, WFLT and Debra S. Knapp, CPT, ACE, AFAA

ALL RIGHTS RESERVED. No part of this book may be reproduced in any manner without the express written consent of the publisher.
All inquiries should be made to:
Integrated Health Services – Indy
10320 East 79th Street
Indianapolis, IN 46236

Library of Congress Control Number: 2014942807
ISBN 978-1-939550-12-5
First Edition
Printed in the United States of America

Table of Contents

Acknowledgements vii
About the Authors ix
Disclaimer x
Section 1: Introduction to the Manual 1
Section 2: General Principles 3
Section 3: Equipment 9
Section 4: Multi-focal Exercises 15

    Introduction 15
    Arm Circles 15
    Cats and Dogs 16
    Cross-crawling 18
    Frog 19
    Frog Pullovers 20
    Gravity Drop 21
    Hip Crossover 22
    Hip and Neck Settle 23
    Inline Gluteal Contractions 25
    Prone Abduction and Hamstring Curls with a Strap 26
    Prone Ankle Squeezes 27
    Sit-to-stand 28
    Sitting Floor 29
    Sitting Overhead Extension 32
    Standing Wall Clock 34
    Standing Windmill 35

- Static Ankle Squeezes ... 36
- Static Back ... 37
- Static Back Pullbacks ... 40
- Static Wall ... 41
- Static Wall Flexion ... 43
- Superman Sequence ... 44
- Triangle ... 48
- Wall Presses ... 49
- Wall Sit ... 50

Section 5: Respiration ... 53
- Introduction ... 53
- Fragmented Breathing ... 53
- VersaStep Breathing ... 55

Section 6: The Power of Postural Alignment ... 57
- Introduction ... 57
- Postural Alignment Checklist ... 59
- Common Postural Maladaptations ... 62

Section 7: Restoring or Improving Balance ... 67
- Introduction ... 67
- Kneeling on a BOSU ... 68
- Sitting on a Stability Ball ... 69
- Standing on a BOSU ... 70

Section 8: Foot and Ankle Processes ... 73
- Alternating Heel Toe ... 73
- Dorsi- and Plantar Flexion with a Block in Sitting ... 74
- Foot Circles ... 75
- Heel Cord Lengthening in Supine with a Strap ... 77
- Heel (Calf) Raises ... 78
- Prehensile Feet and Toe Spreading ... 80

Toe Raises Leaning on the Wall 81

Wall Drop 81

Treatment of Foot Symptoms 82

    Muscle Cramps in Feet and Legs 82

    Plantar Fasciitis 83

    Pronated Feet 83

    Shin Splints 84

    Supinated Feet 84

Section 9: Knee Processes 87

Pigeon-toed in Standing 87

Side Lying Tensor Fascia Latae (TFL)/Iliotibial 88

    Tract (IT) Release with VersaStep 88

Side Lying Unilateral Knee Extension 89

Sitting Floor with Leg Lifts 90

Soft Tissue Knee Balance 91

Section 10: Hip/Low Back Stability Processes 95

Asymmetrical Horizontal Roll 95

Bilateral Horizontal Roll 96

Bilateral Horizontal Roll in Frog 97

Bridging 98

Hip Flexor Release with VersaStep 100

Medial and Lateral Hip Stabilization 101

Pelvic Tilts with VersaStep 103

Section 11: Lower and Middle Thoracic Processes 107

Counter Stretch 107

Crocodile 108

Half Bridging 109

Prone Body Gliding 110

Prone Thoracic Muscular Reeducation 111

Sitting Thoracic Rotation 112

Section 12: Upper Thoracic/Shoulder Processes 115

Backwards Shoulder Rolls 115

Double Leg Drop with Mini-windmills 116

Shoulder and Arm Glide Progression 118

Snow Angels 119

Standing Thoracic Rotation with Extended Arm 121

Sternum Tilts with Double VersaStep 122

Upper Spinal Floor Twist 123

Walking Arm and Shoulder Presses 124

Section 13: Upper Extremity Processes 127

Introduction 127

Back Stroking on the Stability Ball 127

Unilateral Pullover with Resistance 129

Horizontal Unilateral Triceps 130

Section 14: Head/Neck Processes 133

Introduction 133

Head/Neck Clock on VersaStep 133

Static Extension Position 134

Supine Feet-to-Head Release with VersaStep 135

Wall Towels 136

Section 15: Sequences of Exercises for Specific Areas of Function 139

Hip Sequence #1 139

Hip Sequence #2 139

Shoulder Sequence #1 139

Shoulder Sequence #2 139

Scapular Sequence 140

Section 16: Bibliography/References 143

Section 17: Glossary 145

Acknowledgements

We would like to thank Moishe Feldenkrais and Ruthy Alon for their pioneer work in developing somatic movement-based treatment systems and Pete Egoscue for his work in postural alignment and pain management. We appreciate the input and feedback of our clients, families and friends.

About the Authors

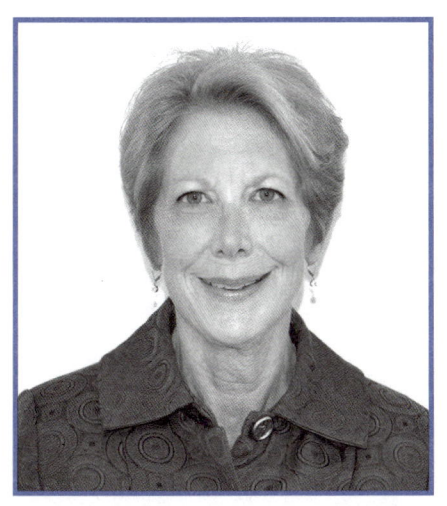

Shereen D. Farber, Ph.D., OTR, FAOTA, BFLT, WFLT is an occupational therapist and neurobiologist. She is a fellow of the American Occupational Therapy Association and is a teacher in Bones for Life and Walk for Life. She was an associate professor of occupational therapy at Indiana University School of Medicine Allied Health Sciences for twenty-five years and has had two private practices, Ortho-Neuro-Rehab Services, treating people with chronic pain and movement disorders in Indianapolis, Indiana since 1974 and Canine Equine Rehab Services where she treats dogs and horses with movement disorders or pain since 1978. Dr. Farber has lectured on neurorehabilitation all over North America. She is the author of numerous articles and texts.

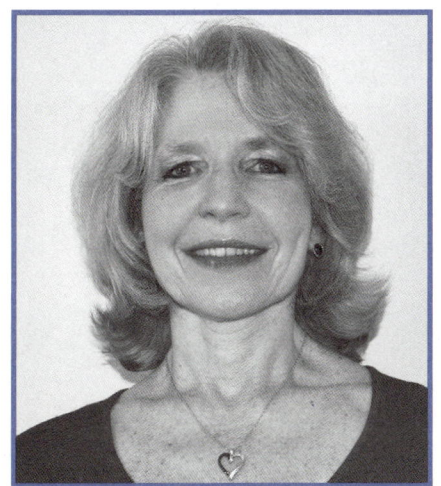

Debra S. Knapp, CPT, ACE, AFAA, Certified Egoscue Posture, Alignment & Pain Management Specialist has been a teacher, coach and personal trainer for over thirty-five years. She has been certified by the American Council on Exercise, the Aerobics and Fitness Association of America, and Egoscue University. She has authored articles on health, wellness and nutrition for various publications. Deb has given numerous presentations at coaches and leadership conferences. Currently, she is a consultant and trainer for the Indiana Parkinson's Foundation.

Health Disclaimer Any participant having fused bones or joints needs to use care in application of the processes in this book. Results may vary depending on the status of soft tissue and the complexity of dysfunction. Anyone having recent surgery or an ongoing chronic condition should consult a physician before starting an exercise program. Ultimately, you are responsible for monitoring your body while using this book as a guide.

Section 1: Introduction to the Manual

Initially, we came together as client (Shereen) and trainer (Deb), both having backgrounds in pain management and over eighty years of combined experience in clinical application. We soon became a treatment team seeing individuals with postural problems. Our training differs, allowing us to merge a multitude of ideas and concepts that produce improved methods of addressing pain and innovative restoration procedures that can be utilized by both amateurs and professionals. Our intension was to create a user-friendly manual for the lay public and to expand ideas for health practitioners. Some of these exercises have been adapted from various treatment systems and others are original to our methodology. Our clients emphatically requested that we write and publish our work.

Our exercises serve to reeducate muscles to do their job, restore functionally designed posture, teach the nervous system to modulate muscle tone for the appropriate actions, and improve circulation. Restoration is a process that takes time before reaching full balanced potential. With consistent corrective measures taught in this book executed persistently, you can improve your daily function. You should notice a positive change each time you do a process. Have a spirit and mindset of experimentation and discovery as you work with this material.

Should you experience difficulty or discomfort during an exercise, proceed with caution. As your muscles stretch, and the skeletal system repositions, any discomfort should diminish. However, if you feel pain, that may be a sign that either you have improper alignment or you are forcing range of motion beyond your body's capability. In the muscle reeducation process, you may activate one or more muscles that has been dormant or less than optimally involved in movement. As these muscles become consistently and correctly engaged, you may experience fatigue. It is important that you continue the exercise beyond what is comfortable in order for those muscles to be strengthened within a functional pattern.

Power Over Pain Intelligent Fitness for the Amateur and Professional

Start with the Multi-Focal section of the manual in order to maximize your time and outcome. The exercises in this section are designed to provide relief to the body as a whole. You may choose to do any individual exercise and still produce a positive result. The remainder of the manual is organized in regions from the feet to the head. If you are attempting to remedy a pain in a specific region of your body, remember that the location of the pain may not necessarily be the source of the problem. If you do not get relief after performing body region specific exercises, you need to refer to the Multi-Focal section of the manual.

The Sequence section of the book lists groups of exercises in a specific order so that your body's response to an individual process will prepare you for the remainder of the sequence. You may also notice an improvement in your sense of balance and experience a reduction in pain and/or tightness.

Remember, any exercise in the manual has the potential to influence other body regions, either directly or indirectly. This is especially true if exercises are executed while using ideal alignment. All processes used in this manual have been individually and group tested with our clients.

Section 2: General Principles

Introduction: Three movement pioneers have influenced our ideas, work, and material. We praise the foundational work in movement therapy and somatic education of Dr. Moise Feldenkrais and Ruthy Alon and the posture and muscular reeducation efforts of Pete Egoscue. Our frame of reference continues to evolve but currently consists of the core beliefs we have outlined in this section regarding function, optimal movement, and intervention. Each of the elements listed below is integral to our philosophical base and represents the facets we consider when evaluating clients and developing action plans. Our biomechanical orientation of the musculoskeletal system forms the basis of our means for intervention. We also consider a developmental hierarchy of skill acquisition when planning client programs. Comprehending our rationale will assist you in understanding biomechanical issues and selecting appropriate exercises.

Awareness: In order for change to take place in your status, there must be an element of consciousness. You must take inventory of your posture, habits, discomforts, daily routines, and environment. You cannot identify and change what you do not acknowledge. You must also take personal responsibility for active intervention so that you can experience empowerment as you back away from your pain patterns and substitute and create healthy new movement.

Balance: In any system that functions perfectly, balance prevails. There is an interrelationship between the parts of a system that promotes equilibrium. For example, the biceps and triceps muscles are reciprocal and must be balanced for your arm to function normally and align properly at your side. Pairs or groups of muscles throughout the body work in this manner. Ideal muscular balance allows an individual to prevent falls, create stability, change direction efficiently, and maximize postural alignment. Muscle imbalances are extremely common and can produce postural misalignment, dysfunction, and pain. If a muscular pair remains unbalanced for a prolonged period of time, one of the pair shortens and tightens while the opposing muscle lengthens and weakens (stretch weakness). So many of us sit at our computers for hours without stopping to get up and move. Most likely, the majority of us have tight chest muscles and weakened muscles in the upper and mid back, creating a muscle imbalance that leads to rounded upper back and forward head and shoulders. As you progress through this book, you will discover many simple and effective exercises you can use to remedy muscle imbalance while taking your breaks.

Bilateral Versus Unilateral: As a result of our everyday routines and our genetics, we develop a dominant body side or region which we often overuse, creating repetitive strain injury and muscular imbalance. If you always train bilaterally, working both sides at the same time, you are unaware of the discrepancy between body sides and any weakness or compensation you have developed. Training unilaterally strengthens weak regions, such as a non-dominant side, and mandates stability on the opposing side. We encourage you to develop skill in your non-dominant side to promote increased stability.

Breathe: Human life cannot exist without respiration, yet many times when you learn a new skill or are lifting weights, you hold your breath. Holding your breath can disrupt the coordination and rhythm of the exercise while disproportionally increasing your blood pressure. In actuality, breathing deeply makes the new skill easier to do or the weight easier to lift.

Change: In general, the human body adapts best to gradual change in most areas of function. We recommend you make changes over time by slow, consistent repetition, allowing you to have more control in the process. In contrast, rapid, forceful movement brings in momentum and reduces control. There are changes that occur following any exercise; however, you can produce long-term results if you maintain an active, balanced exercise program coupled with an awareness of what you are doing and of your postural alignment.

Conditioning: By doing a planned and balanced exercise program with variety, over time you can reduce the amount of effort and demand on your body. In other words you can make yourself more fit. By becoming more fit, all of your body's systems work more efficiently, even your immune system.

Section 2: General Principals

Core: Your core is made up of your entire body minus your extremities. Core is foundational to posture, strength, stability, and functional movement. Core muscles serve to protect organ systems, provide an axis of support, improve upright posture, maximize athletic skill, and distribute gravitational stress effectively. We recommend you work in multiple and combination planes of movement in order to optimize your core.

Dynamic Tension: Dynamic tension is defined as a state of tension or pull that exists between the front surface and back surface of the body. This tension must be balanced in order to promote the movements of extension and flexion in a healthy manner (Egoscue, 1998).

Endurance: Endurance is defined as the ability to withstand demand for an extended period of time. It requires the stamina to sustain a physical activity for a sufficient period of time to accomplish the task. Endurance also refers to both cardiovascular and pulmonary durability as well as musculoskeletal resilience. For example, can you climb several flights of stairs without exhaustion?

Neutrality: Within the range of motion of any joint, there is a point called *neutral* at which the tension is balanced on all sides without stress. You need to go into a neutral position prior to initiating a movement or exercise. For example, before lifting your arms, the shoulder region should be neutralized by lifting the sternum up against gravity and pulling the shoulder blades down and back toward midline. This is particularly important if you have tightness in the chest muscles and at the front of your shoulders. The state of neutrality decreases stress and pain, increases range of motion and stability, and improves the quality of movement. Lack of ability to go into neutral creates dysfunctional and compensation patterns. Once dysfunction is imposed on a normal musculoskeletal system, it loses the ability to return to neutral and to optimize movement. Unless this dysfunction is addressed, the quality of movement and range of motion will only decrease.

Nutrition: The quality of your nutrition influences all systems within the body and is actually a determining factor of good health in general. There are numerous resources available to advise you regarding the ideal ratio of protein, carbohydrates, and fats; ideal caloric intake based on body type and activity level; understanding product labels; amount of hydration necessary, etc. While nutrition is beyond the scope of this book, it is well worth independent study.

Optimal Wellness: When an individual has a balanced awareness of mind/body/spirit, wellness can flourish.

Overflow: Overflow is extraneous movement, often occurring when learning new skills or reeducating new muscular patterns. It can be expressed as a stronger muscular contraction than what is required for that specific pattern or as extra movement taking place outside of the pattern being stimulated. Overflow is maladaptive and if you allow its expression continually, you will not develop the skill or pattern. When overflow happens, you need to simplify the pattern by breaking it down into smaller movement segments, even isolating weaker muscles.

Patterns of Dysfunction: Following trauma, extensive sedentary lifestyle, or repetitive use of compensatory patterns, people often demonstrate lockstepped movement. They cannot isolate individual muscles or muscle groups at least in some part of their bodies. Instead, they unconsciously fire whole patterns of movement that often include flexion, internal rotation, pronation, adduction, and thoracic offset. If you have such dysfunctional patterns, you need to expand your awareness of your inability to isolate a specific movement and then reduce the demand and complexity of the pattern until the desired performance is achieved. Once you can isolate an individual movement, be aware that the individual muscles may fire more slowly at first. With repeated practice of isolated movement, you can achieve efficiency of movement. Occasionally, old patterns, even those newly integrated, can reemerge when your body is stressed. This may be a result of deep fascial binding that is residual from the prior pathological pattern and will require the intervention of a health care professional who works with fascia.

Postural Pain Management: When you first notice even subtle signs of postural pain, discomfort resulting from poor postural alignment, do not ignore the pain. Don't wait for the pain to worsen. Make time to tackle the problem by doing one or more of the exercises listed in the Multi-focal Section of this manual. It is important to note that the source of pain is not necessarily the site of the problem. By addressing the body as a whole, you will dissipate or eliminate the discomfort. Beyond that, you need to heighten your awareness and correct or change dysfunctional postural patterns as you recognize them. Postural pain will change if you change faulty biomechanics.

Preparation Before Performance: Make sure you have the prerequisite performance elements mastered prior to undertaking more complex or difficult skills. For example, if you decide to add running to your exercise routine, you will need proper heel strike, appropriate stride length, no hip rotation, good hip extension, minimal torso rotation, and correct arm swing. Lack of one or more of these elements can lead to pain or injury because running triples the demand on joints, and compensation patterns will gradually emerge leading to dysfunction over time. A better choice in this case would be to add walking in addition to addressing your specific postural and biomechanical problems. Walking is easier to control and requires less amplitude and frequency of movement, reducing joint impact.

Sedentary Lifestyle: In today's technology-based society, many are continuously consulting smart phones, e-book readers, computers, and game-boys instead of participating in active daily lifestyles. The result is de-conditioned and obese individuals and children who use fine motor movements but lack gross motor skill. We are seeing clients who lack range of motion, strength, endurance and who are in excessive flexion, internal rotation, and pronation. They have a variety of pain issues and repetitive strain problems. Their routine includes sitting for hours without awareness of their postures or work environments. We advocate balancing our lives to include daily exercise and disconnecting from technology long enough to remember how to socially interact. We as a society are losing our ability to move effectively and efficiently. Have you decreased your face-to-face communication? Maybe that is the first exercise you should attempt.

Stability/Mobility: Characteristics of stability include: optimal joint loading, neutrality, ideal center of gravity, and natural base of support. Stability is directly related to ideal postural alignment. The better your posture, the more able you are to manage challenges. A sudden perturbation of balance does not present a problem for one with stable joints. In addition, with good stability, standing on either foot is easy, walking is effortless, hopping or jumping is possible. Mobility in this context refers to the ability to move or flow effortlessly. Each joint has its own specific characteristic movement and range of motion. The body is designed to move by synchronizing all musculoskeletal components. Mobility and stability are reciprocal in nature.

If you have above average flexibility you sacrifice some of your stability. Conversely, if you have above average stability, you will demonstrate less mobility. Maintaining an active lifestyle over decades is essential to sustaining your stability and mobility. When planning your exercise program, achieving proficient mobility and stability should be primary goals.

Straighten Before Strengthen: Aligning your body should be the first step of any exercise program. If you initiate a strengthening program prior to addressing postural issues you are setting yourself up for injury and dysfunction. Any aches or pains may indicate the need to reassess posture, form, and technique. We do not advocate pushing through pain.

Working from the Midline Out: When you are addressing core musculature and stability, you are primarily working the midline muscles. It is important to understand that activation of the midline must come before effectively stimulating peripheral muscles. Midline muscles serve as a solid base of support for use of extremities.

Whole Body View, Analysis of Isolated Components, Post-comparison: Typically, when we see clients for consultation, we observe them from a postural and functional standpoint. We note such things as postural alignment and overall function. The purpose is to gain insight into their pain and obstacles. We then go through a systematic analysis of components including medical and nutritional history, gait, transitional movements, soft tissue balance, range and quality of motion, pain, quantity of hydration, lifestyle patterns, etc. As we address areas needing attention, we build on simple well-executed movements leading into patterns, simple to complex. We are more concerned with the quality of movement than the sheer number of repetitions. At the conclusion of each session, we reevaluate the functional picture.

Congratulations, you have managed to navigate through the dry stuff in this book. Remember the principles we outlined above and enjoy your journey to reduce discomfort and gain power over pain!

Section 3: Equipment

All equipment used in this manual can be purchased from one or more of these sources:

Perform Better Sports Catalog
www.performbetter.com
800-556-7464

Power Systems Fitness Equipment Catalog
www.powersystems.com
800-321-6975

Sportsmith Fitness Products
www.sportsmith.com
888-713-2880

Spri Fitness Equipment
www.spri.com
800-222-7774

Therapy Zone
www.therapyzone.com
800-822-2889

When selecting tubing, order a variety of resistance bands. You will need different resistance for large versus small muscle groups, small versus large range of motion, and so on. When ordering a stability ball, the general rule is forty-five centimeters for an individual under five feet in height. For those five feet to five feet five inches order fifty-five centimeters size. For five feet six inches and taller order sixty-five centimeters.

Power Over Pain Intelligent Fitness for the Amateur and Professional

Equipment:

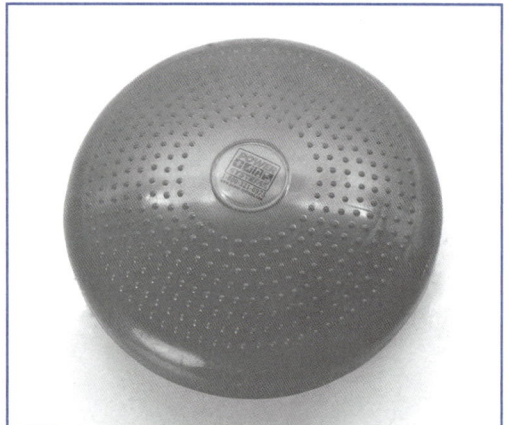

Balance Disc

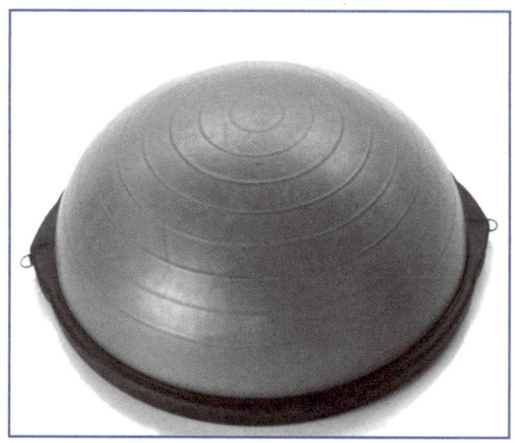

BOSU

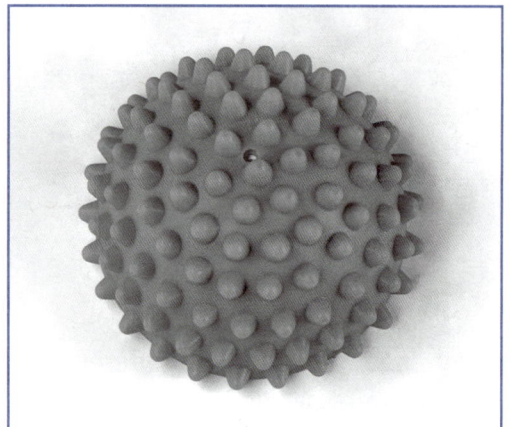

FitPAWS Paw Pods * (This piece of equipment may be used in place of the VersaStep and is slightly smaller.)

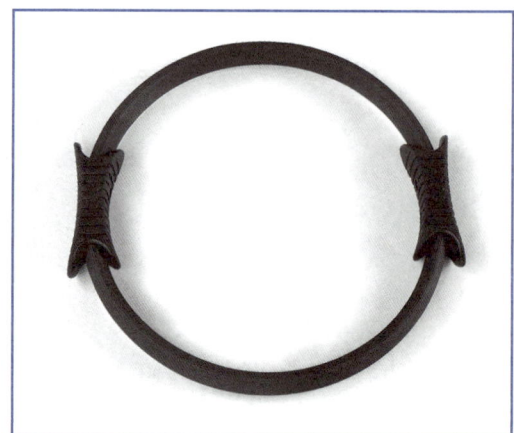

Pilates Ring (optional)

Section 3: Equipment

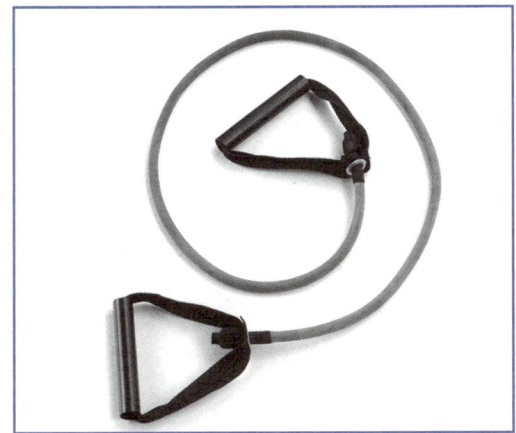

Resistance Tubing

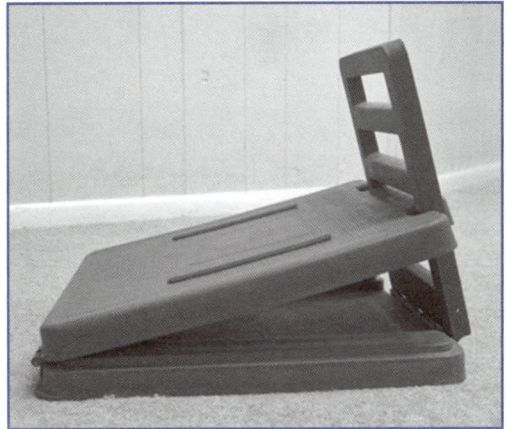

Slant Board or Wedge
(from Therapy Zone)

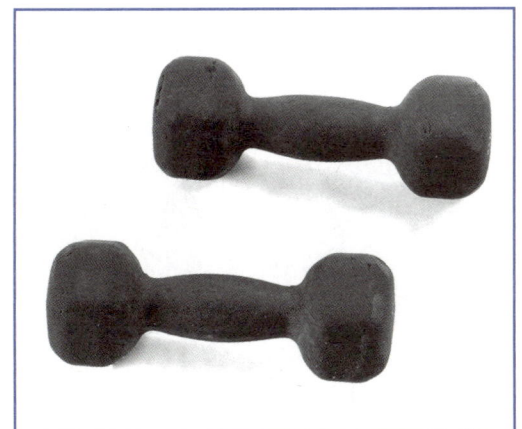

Small Dumbbells

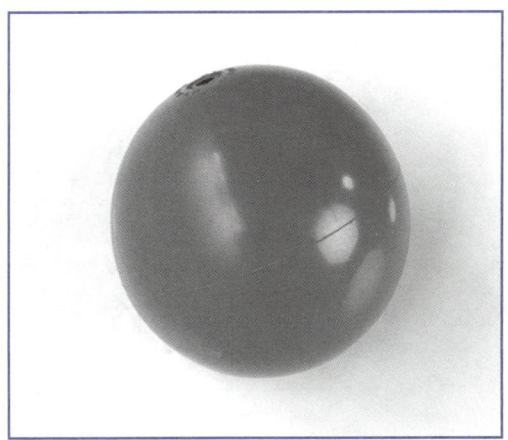

Small Medicine Balls

Power Over Pain Intelligent Fitness for the Amateur and Professional

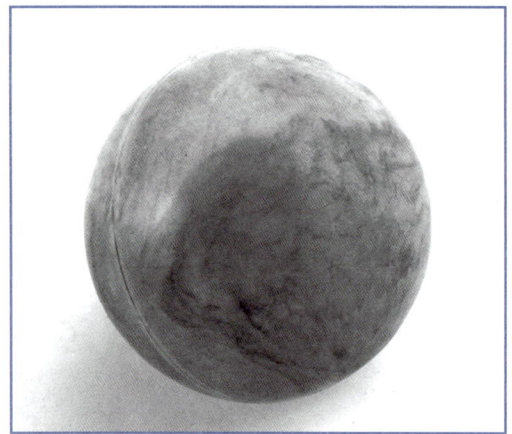

Small Playground Ball

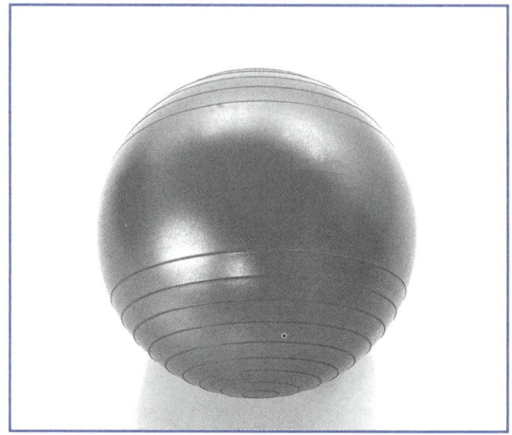

Stability Ball

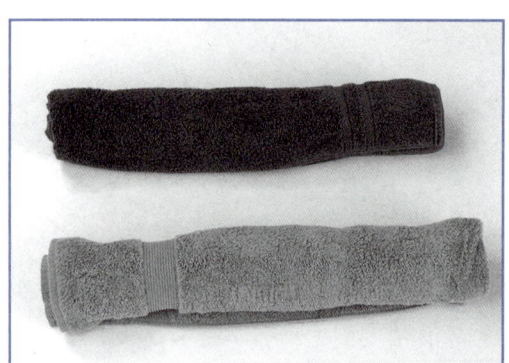

Towels of Various Sizes

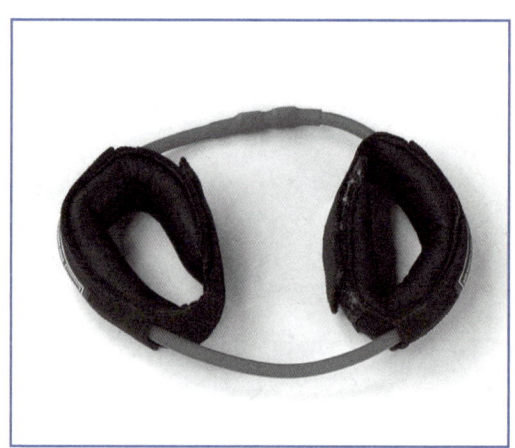

VersaCuff

Section 3: Equipment

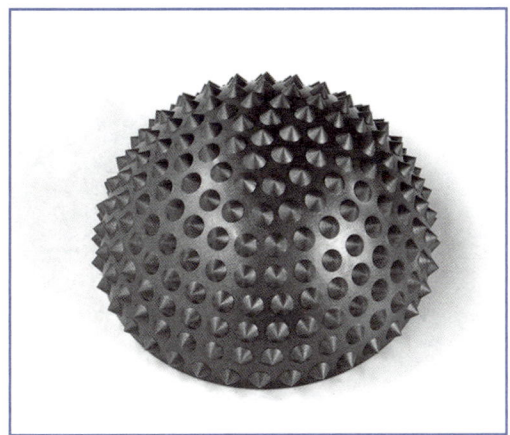

VersaSteps

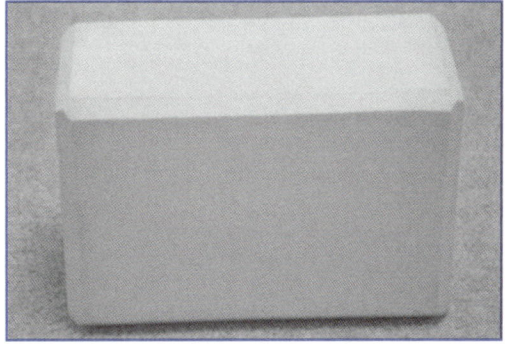

Yoga Blocks

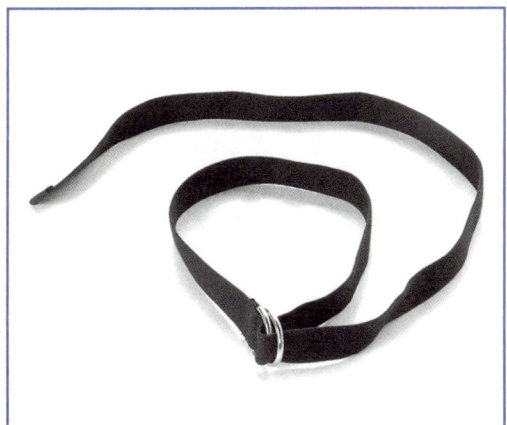

Yoga Strap

Section 4: Multi-focal Processes

Introduction: This section of the book contains exercises that address your entire body helping you use your time more efficiently.

■ Exercise – Arm Circles

Purpose: This exercise serves to strengthen the upper back muscles and modify the dynamic tension and weight distribution throughout the body. It also helps to synchronize the muscles of the shoulder and upper back. If you have head, neck, and shoulder pain, tight chest muscles, weak upper back muscles, forward head, and weak arms, this process is for you.

Contraindications/Precautions: If you have an injury to the rotator cuff you should not do this exercise.

Process:
1. Stand up and assess your posture noting such things as: vertical alignment, position of your shoulders, trunk and hip rotation, forward weight bearing (weight more in the toes and balls of feet versus weight in the heels), and weight evenly distributed.

2. Stand with your shoulders, hips, knees, and ankles all stacked over each other; your head centered over your shoulders.

3. Slightly lift your chest and squeeze your shoulder blades together.

4. Raise your arms to shoulder level with the thumbs forward and palms down.

5. Begin circling the arms up and forward, making six- to eight-inch circles. Make sure you are engaging your upper back, midback, and

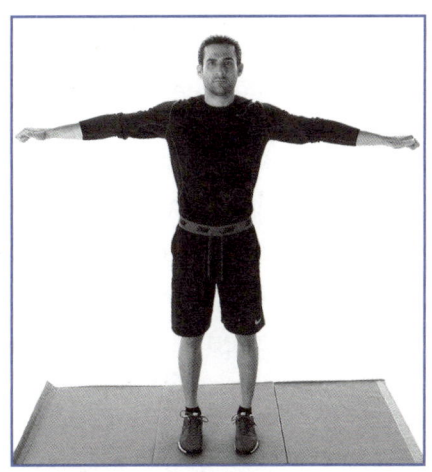

Arm Circles - Process 4

shoulder muscles so that they are working together. Work up to thirty to forty repetitions.

6. Rotate the arms so that the palms are upward and thumbs face backward. Circle the arms up and backward, making six- to eight-inch circles while simultaneously contracting muscles of the upper and mid back and shoulders. Work up to thirty to forty repetitions. *Note: this exercise can also be done in sitting.*

7. Reassess your posture.

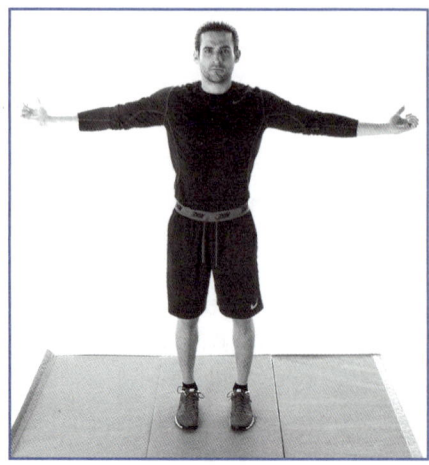

Arm Circles - Process 6

■ Exercise – Cats and Dogs

Purpose: This exercise bilaterally reeducates all load-bearing joints including upper extremities and improves the transition of the entire spine from flexion to extension. It also facilitates evacuation of the bowel, thus positively affecting mood and energy level.

Contraindications/Precautions: If you have had recent wrist or hand surgery, do this exercise on your knees and forearms instead of hands and knees. If you have had recent knee replacement surgery, consult your physician.

Process:

1. Assess any tightness or discomfort and disparity between your right and left side. Rate from one to ten with ten being the most uncomfortable or having the most inequality between body sides.

2. Assume all fours position with knees under the hip joints and hands under the shoulder joints. The distance between the hands should be consistent with the space between the knees. Make sure you do not hyperextend your elbows.

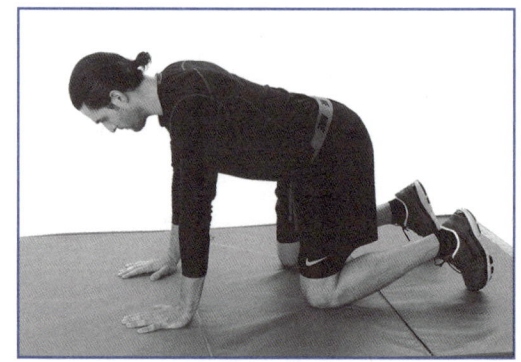

Cats and Dogs - Process 2

Section 4: Multi-focal Processes

3. The cat movement can be compared to a Halloween black cat with the head down and eyes directed toward your knees. Shorten the muscles on the belly side of your body, pulling the hips toward the face, using the lower abdominals. Don't push the hips forward with the gluteal muscles. Be sure to separate your shoulder blades.

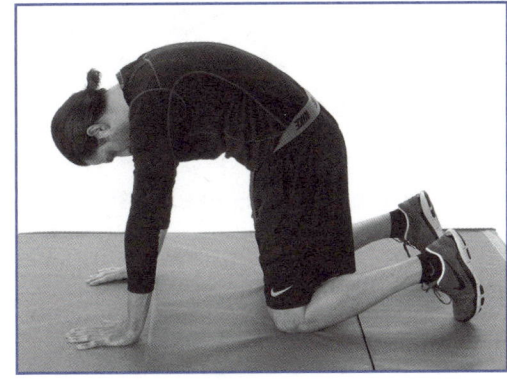
Cats and Dogs - Process 3

4. The dog movement consists of raising the head, pulling the shoulders downward toward your hips and inward toward the spine. Shorten the muscles of the low back, reversing the arch of your spine.

5. As you move smoothly between cat and dog, make sure you keep your arms straight without hyperextension at the elbows. Maintain equal weight distribution on the hands and knees.

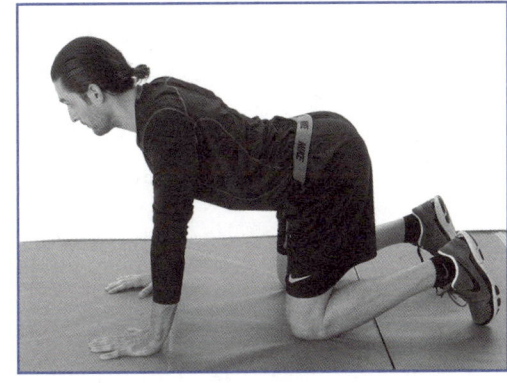
Cats and Dogs - Process 4

Movement between positions should be strictly vertical. **Do not** shift your weight back to your knees when moving to the cat position. Repeat ten to twelve times.

6. Reassess your discomfort and disparity between body sides.

Modification:

Twisted Cats and Dogs: Once you have completed the recommended ten to twelve repetitions of Cats and Dogs, remain on all fours in the cat position and shift the weight in the hips to the left. Look under your left arm toward the outside of your left hip. Hold this position for one minute. Repeat this movement to the right and hold for one minute. Repeat both sides if necessary.

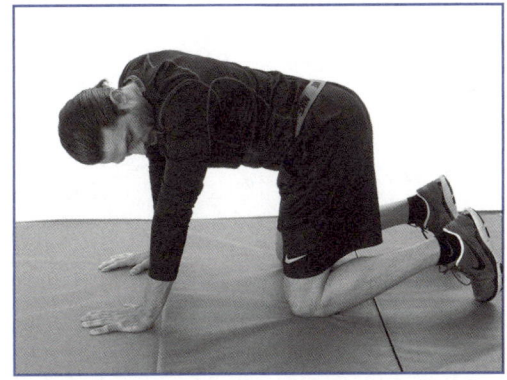
Twisted Cats and Dogs

■ Exercise – Cross-crawling
(Adapted from Egoscue Method, 2001-2003)

Purpose: This exercise reeducates the gait pattern for those who have rotation, poor alignment, and/or muscular compensation. If you have foot, knee, hip, or shoulder pain, do this exercise.

Equipment: Circular tube with VersaCuffs optional.

Contraindications/Precautions: None

Process:

1. Gait assessment: Have someone video you walking toward and away from the camera as well as from each side. Take note of your foot position, length of stride, arm swing, symmetry, coordination, and efficiency of movement. Notice also if you have any hip or trunk rotation, dropping of hip or shoulder during gait, and if your head is centered on your shoulders.

2. Position yourself on your back with legs straight and aligned with your hip joints and your feet parallel and toes pointing straight up. Your arms should be at your sides, palms down.

3. Lift your right knee so that it is over the right hip and the right heel is aligned with your right sits bone. Raise the left arm over your head, keeping the arm straight and close to your head. Simultaneously return both extremities to their start position.

4. Raise your left knee so that it is over the left hip and the left heel is aligned with your left sits bone. Raise the right arm over your head, keeping the arm straight and close to your head.

5. Simultaneously return both extremities to their start position.

6. Alternate #3 and #4 patterns until you feel comfortable with the Cross-crawling pattern.

7. Reassess your gait pattern by a second video taping of you walking toward and away from the camera and from each side.

Modification:

A. In #5 above, you returned each arm and leg set to start position. Instead, do left arm-right leg and then switch to right arm-left leg without returning to the start position. This produces a continuous Cross-crawling pattern that helps influence the quality of your gait. If while doing this modification, you experience strain in your low back, go back to doing the pattern as described in the exercise above.

B. You can use a circular tube with cuffs around the ankles for added resistance while doing this pattern. Make sure you are experiencing equal resistance on both sides.

■ Exercise – Frog

Purpose: This exercise helps to gain range of motion at the hip, decreases hip rotation, and increases sacroiliac joint stability. It also indirectly affects the torso by decreasing rotation and reducing excessive involuntary muscle contraction in the lower and thoracic back.

Contraindications/Precautions: If you have had recent hip or knee surgery, consult your physician before doing this exercise.

Process:

1. Lie on your back, arms out to the side with your palms up and open. Bring your feet together at midline so that your soles are touching, heel to heel and toes to toes. Feet should be positioned a comfortable distance from your torso. Allow your knees to fall outward.

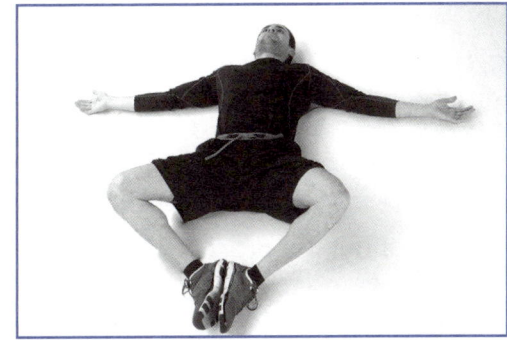

Frog - Process 1

2. Assess the amount of tightness in your legs, hips, torso, shoulders and neck.

3. Remain in this position three to five minutes until you notice decreased tightness in your hips and knees.

Modification: Frog can be done using a VersaStep. The VersaStep should be placed flat side down, centered above the gluteals and tailbone on the body midline. If the textured side of the VersaStep is too uncomfortable, place a small towel over it.

Power Over Pain Intelligent Fitness for the Amateur and Professional

■ Exercise – Frog Pullovers
(Adapted from Egoscue Method, 2001-2003)

Purpose: This exercise helps to gain range of motion at the hip, removes hip rotation, and increases sacroiliac joint stability. With pullovers, you are changing the dynamic tension in your torso by bilaterally reeducating the muscles of the upper and mid back.

Contraindications/Precautions: If you have had recent hip or knee surgery, consult your physician before doing this exercise.

Process:

1. Lie on your back, arms out to the side with your palms up. Bring your feet together at midline so that your soles are touching, heel to heel and toes to toes. Feet should be positioned a comfortable distance from your torso. Allow your knees to fall outward.

2. Assess the degree of tightness you experience in your legs, hips, torso, shoulders, and neck after assuming the frog position.

3. Remain in this position several minutes until you notice decreased tightness in hips and knees.

4. Add pullovers by lifting arms and hands directly over your shoulder joints with elbows in extension.

5. Lower your arms over your head as far as you can without bending at the elbows. Make sure you keep your hands close enough for the thumbs to be able to touch and the elbows extended throughout the process.

6. Bring the arms back over the chest as in #4. Repeat pullovers slowly for at least two minutes or until you feel reduced tightness in the shoulders and torso.

Note: If your elbows begin to bend while bringing them over your head, limit your range of motion to what you can do with the arms straight.

7. Reassess

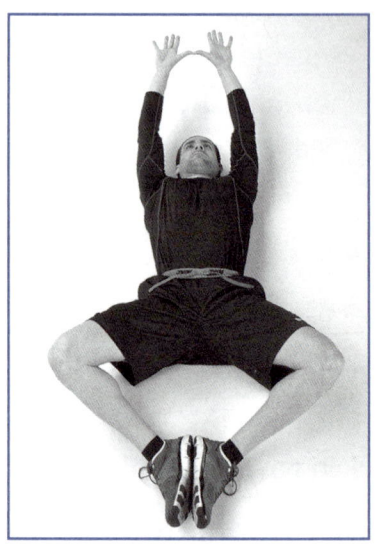

Frog Pullovers - Process 5

Section 4: Multi-focal Processes

Modifications:

A. Place a strap or VersaCuff at the wrists and push outward during the pullover process.

B. Place a resistance tube in your hands, or a VersaCuff on your wrists and pull apart at the top of the pullover. Bring your arms back to parallel before returning arms back over chest.

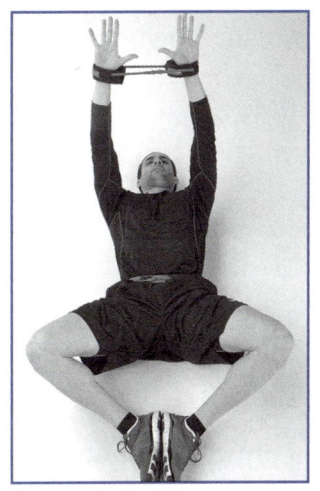

Frog Pullovers - Modification B

■ Exercise – Gravity Drop
(Adapted from Egoscue Method, 2001-2003)

Purpose: This exercise realigns the body from feet to head while correcting dynamic tension and improper joint loading. It also elongates the heel cords.

Equipment: Stairs with handrails or a step bench (located near a wall to hold onto)

Contraindications/Precautions: None

Process:

1. While standing, assess your posture noting such things as: vertical alignment, position of your shoulders, trunk and hip rotation, forward weight bearing (weight more in the toes and balls of feet versus weight in the heels), and weight evenly distributed.

2. Wearing athletic shoes, place feet on a stair or step bench so that the heels remain free and unsupported. Place both hands on railings or stationary objects.

3. Align your body directly over the unsupported heels making sure you do not lean forward. Also make sure your head is centered directly over your shoulders. Allow your heels to drop and then remain in this position for at least five minutes or until you feel the changes in your legs and as far up as your shoulders, neck, and head.

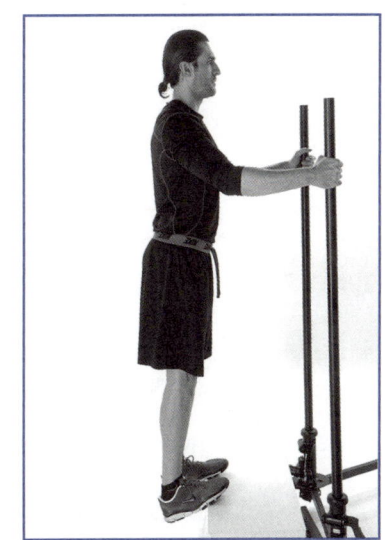

Gravity Drop - Process 3

Power Over Pain Intelligent Fitness for the Amateur and Professional

4. Step down off stairs or step bench and reassess your posture.

Note: If you do not have good body awareness, you may want to do this process in front of a mirror, or have a friend take photos of you, from both front and side views.

■ Exercise – Hip Crossover
(Adapted from Egoscue Method, 2001-2003)

Purpose: This exercise is designed to increase range of motion at the hips, torso, shoulders, and neck. It also may change the baseline position of the knees.

Contraindications/Precautions: If you have had recent hip surgery, consult your physician before doing this exercise.

Process:

1. Assess the tightness in your hips, back, neck, and shoulders. Rate the tightness from one to ten with ten being extremely tight.

2. Lie supine with bent knees, heels in line with sits bones and arms at shoulder level, palms up.

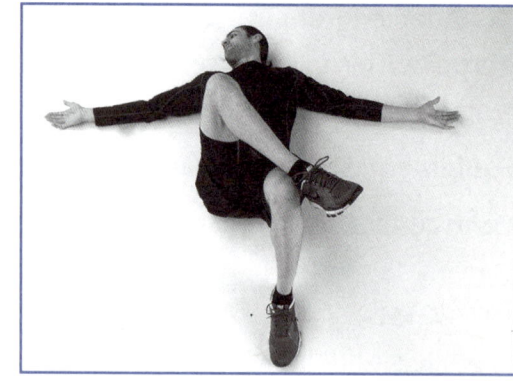
Hip Crossover - Process 3

3. Without moving your left foot, knee, and hip, cross your right ankle over your left knee and then turn your head so that you are looking at your right hand. Drop both legs to the left as far as your body will allow. Open the right hip and knee as far as you can.

4. Hold at least sixty seconds.

5. Return to supine bent knee position as in #2 and repeat the process on the other body side, holding for at least sixty seconds.

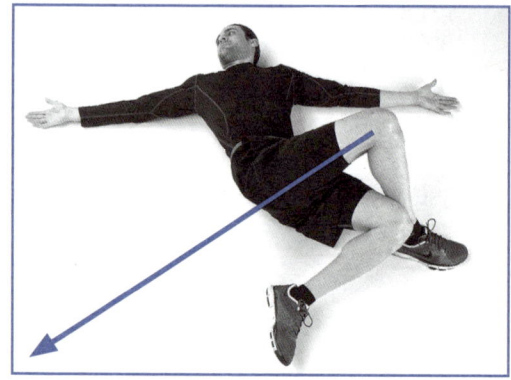
Hip Crossover - Process 3

6. Reassess the tightness in your hips, back, neck, and shoulders.

Section 4: Multi-focal Processes

■ Exercise – Hip and Neck Settle

Purpose: This exercise is designed to address hip rotation and pain in any of the following areas: ankles, feet, knees, pelvic floor, hips, sacroiliac joint, back, shoulders, and neck. The towel helps support the lumbar and cervical spine, low back, and neck muscles, allowing tight muscles to relax. It serves to reeducate the lumbar and cervical curves.

Equipment: Two bath towels, VersaStep, massage ball, or FitPAWS Paw Pods

Contraindications/Precautions: If the neck or low back becomes uncomfortable during the process, unroll the towel(s) to a smaller diameter that is more comfortable.

Process:

1. Start by rating your hip, low back, shoulder, head, neck, and jaw pain levels from one to ten with ten representing the worst pain.

2. Lie on your back and place one towel under the lumbar spine and one under the cervical spine, both positioned perpendicular to the midline of the body. Towels should be rolled tightly, the diameter adjusted based on the amount of pain you are experiencing. The more severe the pain, the smaller the diameter of towel used. Lie in supine with bent knees; your feet should be parallel and in line with sits bones. Allow the hips, shoulders, and neck to settle for up to ten minutes.

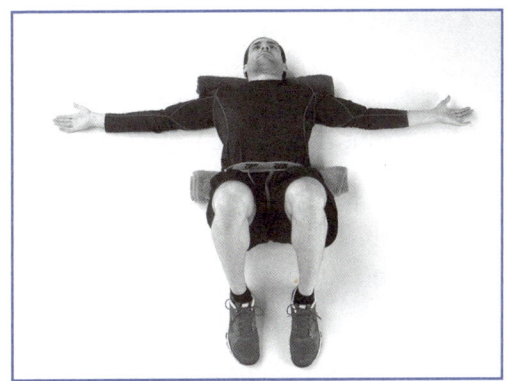

Hip and Neck Settle - Process 2

3. Reassess hip, low back, shoulder, head, neck, and jaw pain.

Modifications:

A. Hip Settle and Hip Drops with VersaStep (or equivalent equipment): After assuming the position of Hip Settle described in #2 above, replace the towel with a small massage ball, FitPAWS Paw

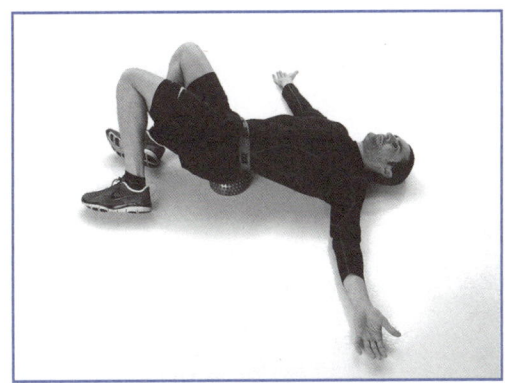

Hip and Neck Settle - Modification A

Pods, or a VersaStep. Position the chosen equipment centered above the gluteals and tailbone on the body midline. Allow the hips to settle around the equipment until you feel your hips drop toward the floor. Initially, it takes approximately ten minutes for the hips to drop. Try side-to-side hip drops, continuing to breathe deeply with each direction change.

B. Hip Settle with Reverse Presses:
After assuming the position of Hip Settle described in #2 above, place your arms in an upright goalpost position. Press elbows, upper arms, and muscles between the shoulders into the floor, making sure the shoulder joint goes backward and close to the floor. Repeat for two minutes. (Egoscue Method, (2001-2003)

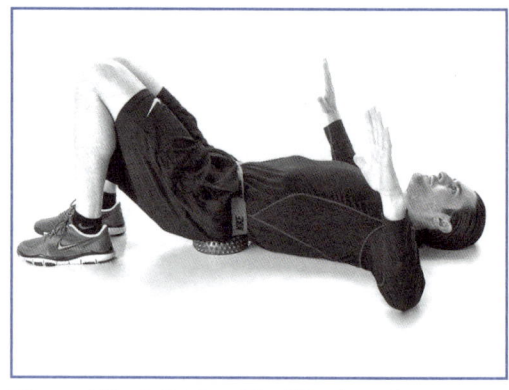
Hip and Neck Settle - Modifications B

C. Hip Settle with Pullovers: After assuming the position of basic Hip Settle described in #2 above, extend your arms above your chest. Keeping your arms close enough so that your thumbs can touch, lower your arms over your head by activating the muscles of your upper and middle back. Limit your range of motion to what you can do with your arms straight. Repeat for two minutes.

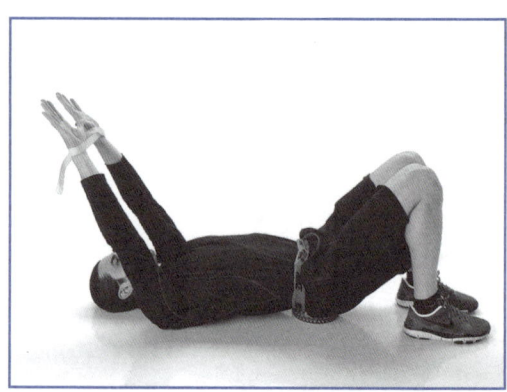
Hip and Neck Settle - Note

Note: Pullovers may also be done with a strap around the wrists; continuing to use upper and mid back muscles, push out against the strap.

Section 4: Multi-focal Processes

■ Exercise – Inline Gluteal Contractions

(Adapted from Egoscue Method, 2001-2003)

Purpose: This process provides vertical and bilateral loading, activates muscles in the posterior chain, and eliminates trunk and hip rotation. It also promotes foot and ankle stability.

Contraindications/Precautions: None

Process:

1. Stand in front of a mirror. Assess your weight distribution and note if you are rotated at hips or trunk. Walk a short distance noting the position of your feet (are they turned outward) and if you feel contractions in the gluteal muscles.

2. Place right heel directly in front of the left toes making sure that both feet face directly forward. Pull your torso upright so that your shoulders are centered over your hips and your head is centered on your shoulders. If you are having trouble maintaining your balance, place one finger on a stationary object located near waist level.

3. Focus your eyes on an object located straight ahead. Lift the sternum and contract the abdominal muscles while keeping the shoulder blades together.

Inline Gluteal Contractions - Process 2

4. Squeeze and release the gluteal muscles without engaging your abdominals or your quads. Continue repetitions for two minutes. For some of you, the longer you sustain this process, the easier it gets while for others, fatigue will ensue during the two-minute period.

5. Repeat the process with the left heel in front of the right toes.

6. Reassess weight distribution, hip, and trunk rotation and changes in your gait and foot position.

■ Exercise – Prone Abduction and Hamstring Curls with a Strap

(Adapted from Egoscue Method, 2001-2003)

Purpose: These two processes done in sequential order provide a powerful tool for diminishing hip, low back, and knee pain. They serve to promote horizontal loading from knees to the head and help to stabilize ankles, knees, hips, and low back. They assist in removal of hip rotation and engage the muscles of the lateral hip and leg. These exercises specifically promote bilateral involvement of the muscles and joints of the low back, hips, and legs and address pain caused by muscle imbalance. Anterior, posterior, medial, and lateral hip engagement are all brought to the forefront in this combination of exercises.

Contraindications/Precautions: For those who are uncomfortable in prone (face down), proceed with caution but understand that doing these exercises will help diminish low back pain and hip flexor tightness.

Process:

1. Rate pain from one to ten with ten being the worst in your ankles, knees, hips, low, middle and upper back. Rate your hip flexor tightness from one to ten with ten being the worst.

2. Lie prone placing a yoga strap around your ankles. Your feet should be approximately six to eight inches apart. Position one hand over the other and lower your forehead onto your hands. Bend your knees to a ninety degree angle and dorsi-flex your feet.

3. Push out against the strap for three to five seconds and release. Ideally, there should be no movement in the torso, hips, or legs. As you continue repetitions, any movement there should decrease. After one to two minutes you should notice less discomfort.

4. Lower your legs for fifteen to thirty seconds and take a few deep breaths in through your nose and out through your mouth.

5. Return to the position described in #2, remembering to dorsi-flex your feet. Push out against the strap and slowly lower your legs to the floor, allowing your toes to touch the surface. Continuing to push out against the strap, engage your

Section 4: Multi-focal Processes

hamstrings (muscles on the back of thighs) and return your legs to a ninety degree angle. During these hamstring curls, you may experience extraneous movement in the lower legs that should decrease with repetition.

6. Continue doing hamstring curls for two-to-three minutes. Note if your hips have changed position so that they are flatter to the floor.

7. Reassess pain in your ankles, knees, hips, low, middle and upper back, and reevaluate your hip flexor tightness.

■ Exercise – Prone Ankle Squeezes
(Adapted from Egoscue, 1998; Egoscue Method, 2001-2003)

Purpose: This process provides horizontal loading from the knees to the head, stabilizes hips and low back; removes hip rotation; and addresses knee, hip, low back, and neck pain. It also reeducates gluteals and hamstrings to work bilaterally.

Contraindications/Precautions: None

Process:

1. Rate pain from one to ten with ten being the worst in knees, hips, low back, and neck. Also note if you have hip rotation.

2. Lie prone placing a two-to-three-inch yoga block or pillow between your feet and ankles. Position one hand over the other and lower forehead onto your hands. Bend the knees to a ninety-degree angle and dorsi-flex your feet

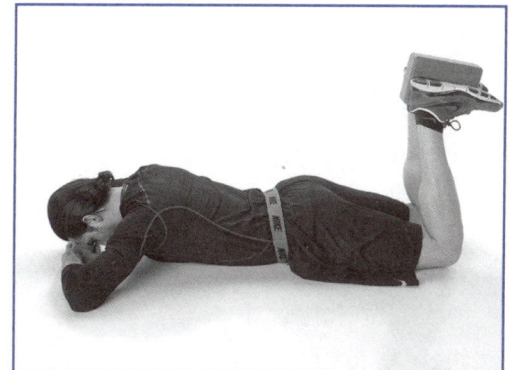

Prone Ankle Squeezes - Process 2

3. Squeeze and release the block or pillow, paying attention to the amount of movement in the legs and hips such as side-to-side wobble. With increased repetition the less movement there should be. Sustain this process for two minutes.

4. Monitor if you feel even weight distribution on the front of your hips. For example, if you do not feel weight on the front of your left hip, bring your left hip downward

toward the floor. The block should be centered with your hips. If you do not feel your gluteals firing, separate the knees slightly and continue the process.

5. Reassess pain in knees, hips, low back, and neck. Compare hip rotation before and after this process.

■ Exercise – Sit-to-stand

(Adapted from Egoscue Method, 2001-2003)

Purpose: Doing this exercise promotes bilateral loading of the feet, knees, and hips without rotation or using the hands to push off. Sit-to-stand improves balance and stability.

Equipment: A bench or stable chair

Contraindications/Precautions: If you have balance issues, make sure you do this process with an additional person to help spot or assist you.

Process:

1. Assess your weight distribution while standing. Is your weight distributed equally on both feet? Do you have balance issues as you move between sitting and standing? Do you have to push off with your hands while transitioning from sit-to-stand?

2. Sit on the edge of a bench or chair with your feet parallel and positioned hip joint distance apart. Place hands behind your head with elbows open and out of your peripheral vision. Keep your torso upright and weight in your heels.

3. Without moving your feet, lean forward slightly, keeping your hips over your heels, and slightly arch your low back. Stand all the way up keeping weight equally on feet and legs.

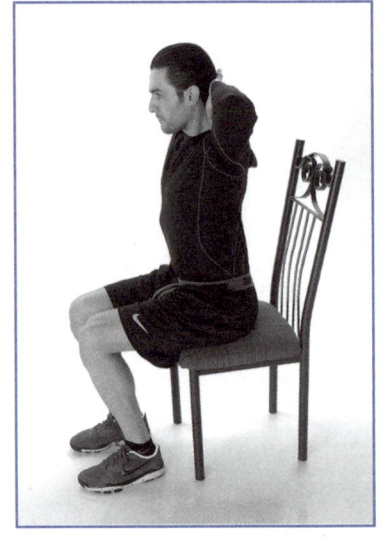
Sit-to-stand - Process 2

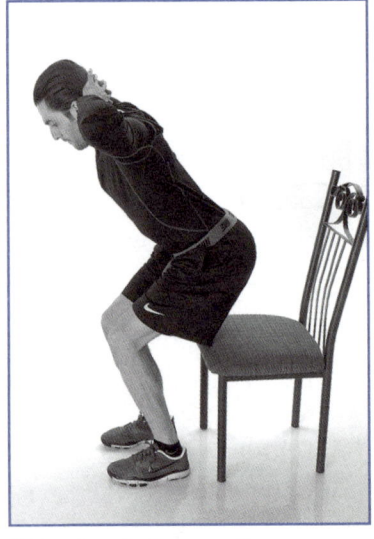
Sit-to-stand - Process 3

Section 4: Multi-focal Processes

4. Slowly lower your hips back to the edge of the bench or chair without moving your feet while maintain the arch in your low back. Remember you are still holding your hands behind your head, and your elbows are open.

5. Repeat steps #3 and #4 until you can do at least twenty-five times without fatigue. You may have to gradually work your way up to this number.

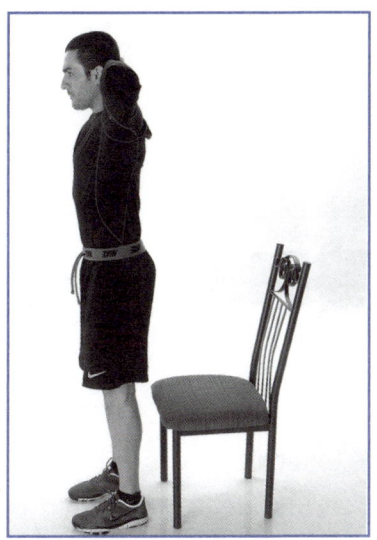
Sit-to-stand - Process 4

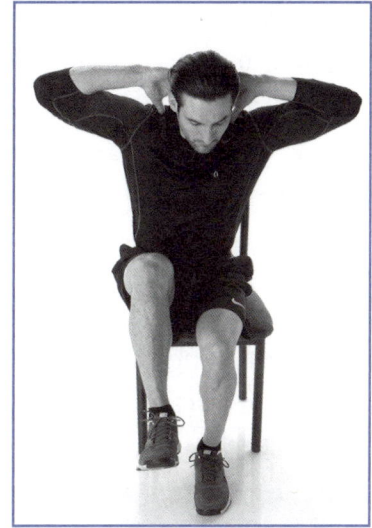
Sit-to-stand - Modification

6. Reassess weight distribution and balance.

Note: Sit-to-stand can also be done with your feet on a BOSU or balance disc.

Modification: This process can be done unilaterally instead of bilaterally.

■ Exercise – Sitting Floor
(Adapted from the Egoscue, 1998; Egoscue Method, 2001-2003)

Purpose: This exercise is designed to reeducate the kinetic chain between the feet, knees, and hips and address dynamic tension of the entire leg, low back, head, neck, and shoulders. You are vertical loading from the head to the hips and horizontal loading from the hips to the feet.

Contraindications/Precautions: If you have sciatic pain, this process may exacerbate the problem. If you have disc dysfunction, the process may make it worse. However, if your sacroiliac joint is out of alignment causing sciatic symptoms, Sitting Floor may help you feel better.

Process:

1. Assess the amount of pain you have in the entire major load-bearing regions (feet, knees, hips, spine, shoulders, and neck). Rate the pain from one to ten with ten being the worst.

2. Find a flat surfaced wall or door; sit and position yourself so that the back of your hips are as close to the wall as possible, legs stretched out in full knee extension and toes pointed toward the ceiling. Head is centered over the shoulders and shoulder blades are pressed into the wall, palms up on your thighs. This is referred to as long sitting.

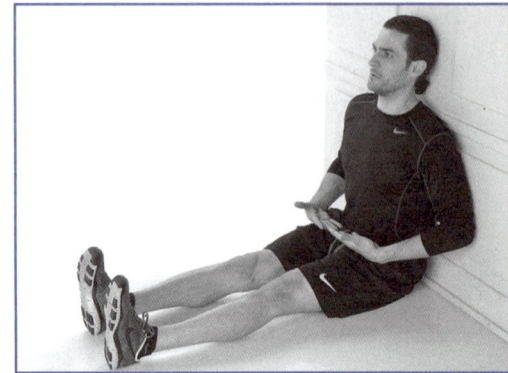

Sitting Floor - Process 2

3. Maintain this position for three to six minutes. If your hamstrings are extremely tight, by doing quad contractions and releases, you will facilitate lower tone and less tightness in the hamstrings.

4. Reassess the load-bearing regions.

Modifications:

A. Sitting Floor with Arm Circles:

1. Assume the Sitting Floor position away from a wall in upright long sitting as described in Sitting Floor # 2. If you cannot sit upright with your legs straight, insert a small towel roll under your knees. Head is centered over the shoulders and shoulder blades are pulled in toward midline. Arms are out to the side with palms down.

2. Make small four-to six-inch-diameter circles with your arms moving in a forward position, making sure you are engaging the muscles between your shoulders. Repeat twenty to forty repetitions.

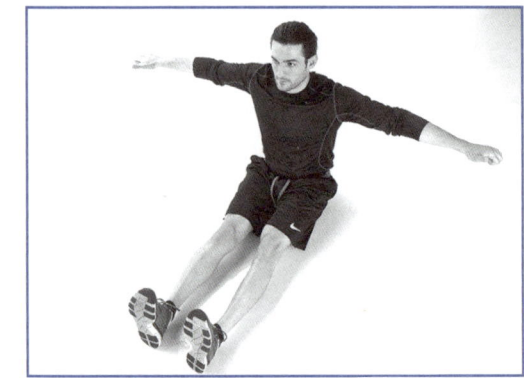

Sitting Floor - Modification A2

Section 4: Multi-focal Processes

3. Rotate the arms so palms are up with thumbs facing backward. Maintain shoulder blades toward midline and head centered on the shoulders.

4. Make small four to six-inch diameter circles with your arms moving in a backward position, making sure you are engaging the muscles between your shoulders. Repeat twenty to forty repetitions.

5. The whole time you are circling your arms, you are also engaging the quads and keeping your toes pointed toward the ceiling.

B. Sitting Floor With Elbow Curls:

1. Assume the Sitting Floor position and maintain for one to two minutes.

2. Bend the elbows with thumbs down and the little fingers up. Place your knuckles against your temples with the elbows open. Keep your quads tight and legs in full extension while maintaining your toes pointing toward the ceiling.

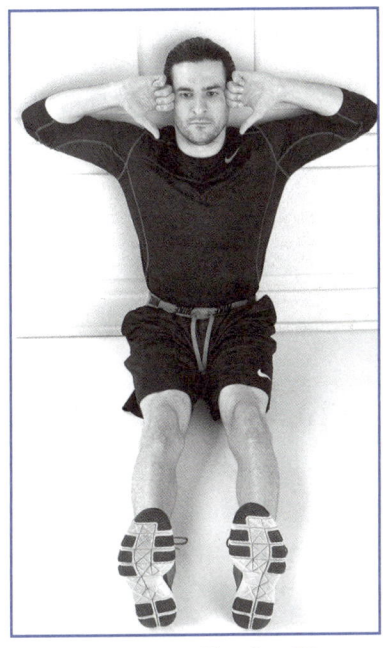
Sitting Floor - Modification B2

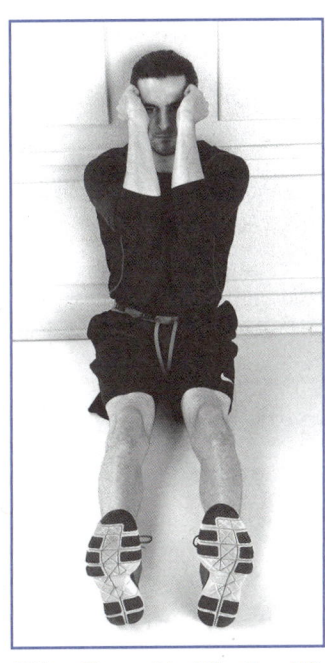
Sitting Floor - Modification B3

3. Keeping your spine on the wall and knuckles against your temples, bring your elbows forward until they touch or until your spine cannot retain contact with the wall.

4. Open your elbows, attempting to touch them to the wall. Concentrate on using the muscles of the upper and midback versus just using your arms to accomplish this action.

5. Repeat #3 and #4 for at least one to two minutes.

Power Over Pain Intelligent Fitness for the Amateur and Professional

C. Sitting Floor with Upright Goalposts:

1. Assume the Sitting Floor position and maintain for one to two minutes.

2. Raise your arms to shoulder height and bend your elbows so that your upper arms are perpendicular to your torso like goalposts. Maintain one to two minutes.

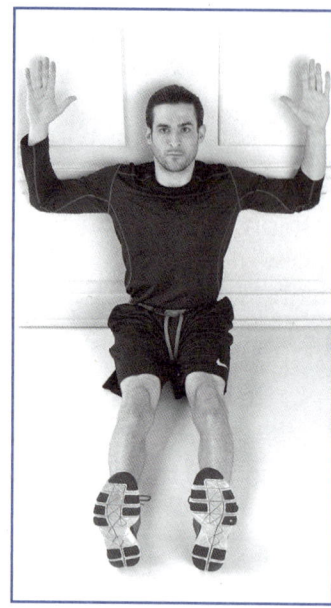
Sitting Floor - Modification C2

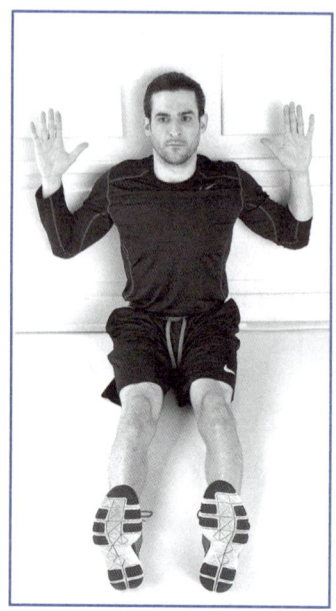
Sitting Floor - Modification C3

3. Keeping your head and the back surface of your arms on the wall as best as you can (start position), pull your elbows slowly downward a few inches and bring your shoulder blades in toward your spine. Return your elbows back to start position and repeat small downward movements each cycle, returning to start position.

■ Exercise – Sitting Overhead Extension
(Adapted from Egoscue Method, 2001-2003)

Purpose: This exercise promotes extension in the cervical, thoracic, and lumbar spine. It also serves to re-center the torso over the hips, removes trunk and hip rotation, and encourages a coordinate pattern of arms, head, and torso.

Equipment: Chair with solid sitting surface

Contraindications/Precautions: Do not force your body into more extension than it is capable. Go slowly and allow time for range of motion to increase gradually. You may experience some dizziness when doing this exercise. It is a common part of the reeducation and repositioning process but should dissipate with repetition.

Section 4: Multi-focal Processes

Process:

1. Assess your postural alignment and weight distribution.

2. Sit on the edge of a chair with your feet parallel directly under your knees. Interlace your fingers, turn them inside out, and extend your arms. If it is too difficult to turn your hands inside out, leave them interlaced with palms facing you. Sit upright in good postural alignment. Keeping your eyes on your fingers, slowly begin to raise your arms until your hands are above your torso. Remember not to force extension and stop when you have reached your limit.

3. Hold this position ideally for one minute and build up to two minutes. If holding this position for one minute is too difficult, then begin by holding fifteen to twenty seconds and build endurance from there.

4. Take a deep breath in through your nose and slowly lower your arms to your lap, continuing to look at your hands throughout the process.

5. Reassess your postural alignment and weight distribution.

Modifications:
This exercise can be done in standing once you have built your tolerance and endurance and can hold the extended position for two minutes. Make sure you do not hyperextend your torso in standing. Instead, keep your shoulders over your hips and allow your head to drop back.

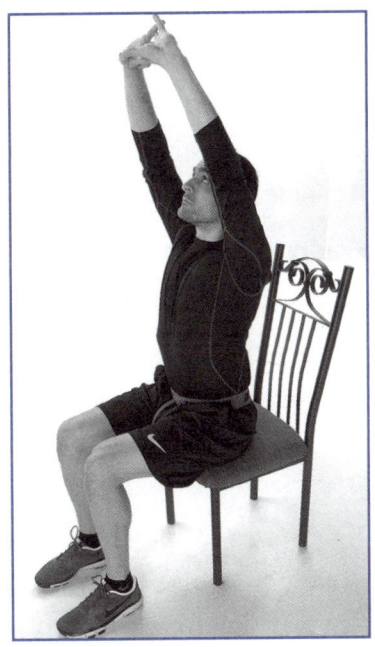

Sitting Overhead Extension - Process 2

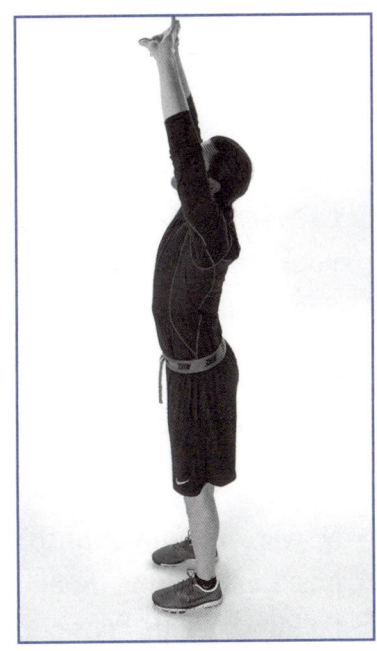

Sitting Overhead Extension - Modification

■ Exercise – Standing Wall Clock
(Adapted from Egoscue, 1998)

Purpose: Standing Wall Clock helps to re-center weight distribution, removes hip and torso rotation, opens and repositions the shoulders, and promotes trunk and hip extension. This exercise is also beneficial for wrist and hand pain.

Equipment: A wall

Contraindication/Precaution: If you have had recent shoulder surgery, consult your physician before attempting this exercise. If you have limited range of motion in the shoulder, proceed with caution and do not force any position.

Process:

1. Observe your alignment in a mirror and notice weight distribution. Are you standing with more weight on one foot and is your weight in your heels or more toward your toes? Are your hips or torso rotated?

2. Face the wall and place your feet in pigeon-toed position. Ideally, your toes should be touching each other and the wall. Check to make sure that each hip is the same distance from the wall. Raise your arms directly over your head with your pinky fingers on the wall and your thumbs pointed back. Hold this position for at least one minute.

3. Lower both arms to ten and two o'clock position. Hold for at least one minute.

4. Now lower your arms to nine and three o'clock position and hold for at least one more minute.
Be mindful if this position causes pain at the elbow. If so, temporarily eliminate this step. Periodically try this step again and add it back into the sequence when there is no pain.

5. Reassess alignment, weight distribution, trunk and hip rotation.

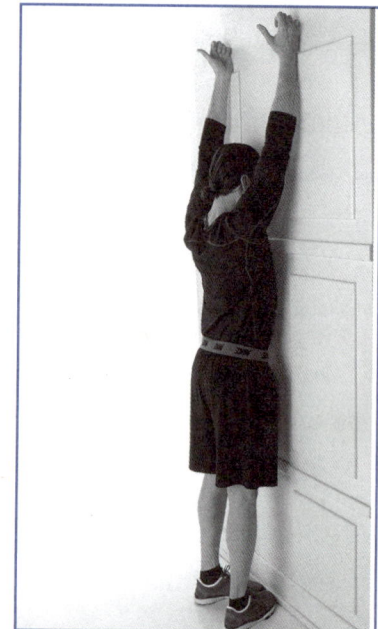

Standing Wall Clock - Process 2

Section 4: Multi-focal Processes

■ Exercise – Standing Windmill
(Adapted from Egoscue Method, 2001-2003)

Purpose: This exercise produces vertical bilateral loading, eliminates rotation, and addresses dynamic tension and lateral flexion and extension. It also redistributes weight equally onto both feet and into the heels.

Equipment: A wall or flat surface large enough to allow for lateral flexion with arms out to the sides at shoulder level

Contraindications/Precautions: None

Process:

1. Observe your alignment in a mirror, especially noting if you have any rotation or asymmetry in your trunk, i.e. one shoulder higher than the other or torso not centered over hips. Is your weight distributed equally over both feet and even from heels to toes?

2. Assume a standing position with your heels against a wall, feet under the hip joints, parallel and facing straight ahead. Your torso should be centered over your hips and your back; shoulders, arms, and head should be touching the wall surface if possible. Arms should be out at shoulder height with palms open.

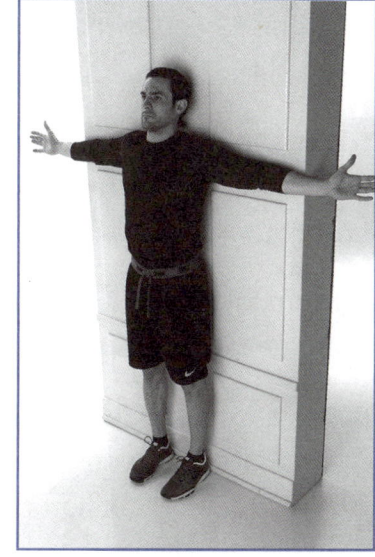
Standing Windmill - Process 2

3. Keeping weight distributed evenly and the hips still; lean to the right while maintaining the trunk, shoulders, arms, and head in contact with the wall; then return to center.

4. Now lean the torso to the left, again keeping the hips still; and the head, shoulders, arms, and back in contact with the wall. Return torso to center.

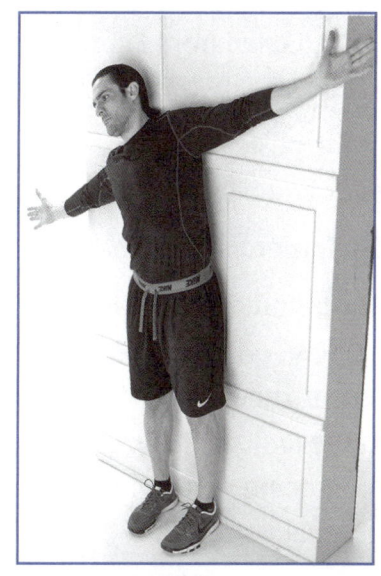
Standing Windmill - Process 3

5. Repeat steps #3 and #4 at least five repetitions to each side. Check the weight distribution in your feet, making sure you are not clawing your toes and that weight is in your heels.

6. Take a small step (four to six inches) to the right with your right foot. Your feet are still perpendicular to the wall but are no longer under your hips.

7. Resume #3 and #4 at least five repetitions to each side.

8. Take another small step to the right. Now your feet should be twelve to sixteen inches apart and continue repetitions as in #3 and #4.

9. Return to your original position as in #2 and resume repetitions to each side as in #3 and #4.

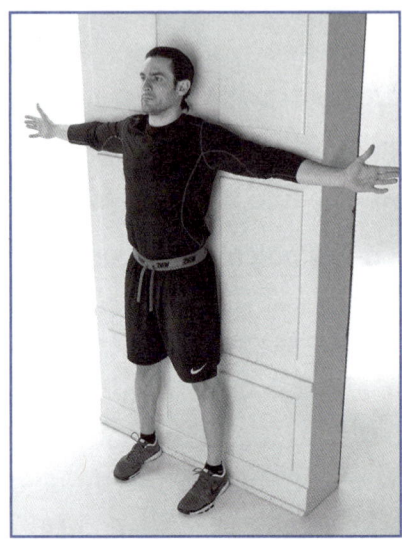

Standing Windmill - Process 6

10. Reassess postural alignment and weight distribution. Do you have less trunk asymmetry and rotation? Has weight distribution changed in your feet?

■ Exercise – Static Ankle Squeezes
(Adapted from Egoscue Method, 2001-2003)

Purpose: This exercise helps eliminate rotation and bilaterally reeducates the muscles of the posterior surface of the body from the head to the heels in order to stabilize the back and hips. It also helps to retrain the load-bearing joints of the upper extremities.

Equipment: A yoga block

Contraindications/Precautions: If you have had recent wrist or hand surgery, do this exercise on your knees and forearms instead of hands and knees. If you have had recent knee replacement surgery, consult your physician. If you have disc dysfunction in the lumbar spine, proceed with caution; discontinue if pain increases in disc region after doing several repetitions. Pain should begin to dissipate after a number of repetitions.

Section 4: Multi-focal Processes

Process:

1. Rate your discomfort in neck, shoulders, back and hips from one to ten with ten being the worst.

2. Assume all fours position with the knees under the hip joints and hands under shoulders. Place a yoga block between your feet and ankles. Walk your hands forward the length of one hand and reposition the torso so that the shoulders are directly over the wrists and hands. Pull shoulders together toward body midline and drop the chin to your chest.

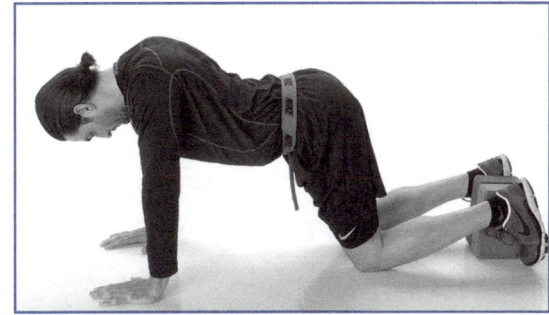
Static Ankle Squeezes - Process 2

3. Slowly squeeze and release the yoga block that you placed between your feet and ankles. Repeat this step for at least two minutes. Remember to engage your triceps so your arms are straight throughout the process.

4. You may experience discomfort in your low back at the start of this exercise. With repetition, the discomfort should dissipate. If you cannot sustain the position for two full minutes, rest and resume the process. Gradually build up your stamina.

5. Reassess your discomfort.

■ Exercise – Static Back

(Adapted from Egoscue, 1998; Egoscue Method, 2001-2003)

Purpose: This exercise decreases hip and trunk rotation as well as allowing the hips to settle into a more neutral pelvis. It horizontally loads the trunk between the pelvis and shoulders.

Equipment: Access to a wall, yoga block, or a chair if you cannot maintain the position described below

Contraindications/Precautions: None

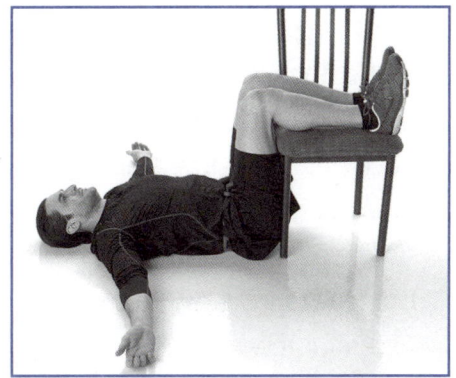
Static Back - Equipment

Power Over Pain Intelligent Fitness for the Amateur and Professional

Process:

1. Assess the discomfort and tightness in your neck, shoulders, torso, low back, hips, thighs, knees, ankles, and feet. Rate these areas from one to ten with ten being the worst.

2. Lie on your back with your knees bent and feet on the wall so that your feet are parallel and hip joint distance apart. Your knees should be directly above your hip joints, forming two ninety-degree angles at the hips and knees. Your trunk should be centered in relationship to your hips and your head should be centered in relationship to shoulders and torso. Your arms should be out to your sides with your palms up.

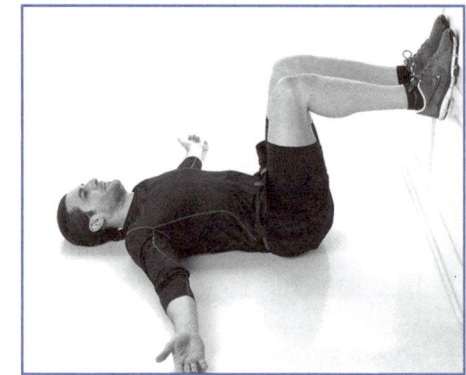

Static Back - Process 2

3. Remain in this position for five to ten minutes, allowing the body to settle. Make sure your feet maintain the original position as described in #2. If you cannot keep your feet on the wall, prop them up on a chair seat.

4. As you are in the Static Back position, note changes as they occur in your areas of tightness and pain. You should experience subtle relaxation over time.

5. Reassess

Modifications:

A. Static Back with Knee Pillow Squeezes:
After assuming the position of basic Static Back described in #2 above, place a yoga block or pillow between the knees and slowly squeeze and release pressure on the block or pillow. Repeat for two minutes.

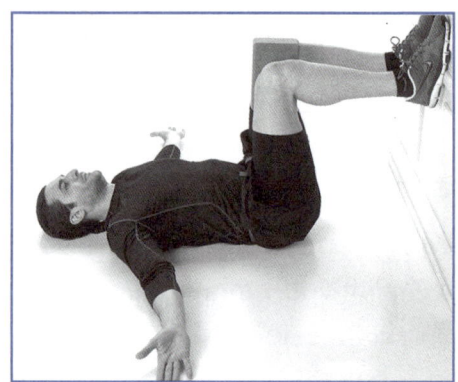

Static Back - Modifications A

Section 4: Multi-focal Processes

B. Static Back with Reverse Presses: After assuming the position of basic Static Back described in #2 above, place your arms in an upright goalpost position. Press elbows, upper arms, and muscles between the shoulders into the floor, making sure the shoulder joint goes backward and close to the floor. Repeat for two minutes. This process can also be done using **Walking Arm and Shoulder Presses**, page 124.

C. Static Back with Pullovers: After assuming the position of basic Static Back described in #2 above, extend your arms above your chest. Keeping your arms close enough so that your thumbs can touch, raise your arms over your head. Limit your range of motion to what you can do with your arms straight. Repeat for two minutes.

D. Static Back Abduction/Adduction: Assume the Static Back position described in #2 above. Drop the knees to midline, making sure your knees are centered. Maintaining contact with the wall, open your knees, allowing the soles of your feet to face each other. Return your knees to midline and again drop your knees open, moving your feet as described above. Continue this process for two to three minutes. This modification adds hip and low back stability by way of internal and external femoral rotation.

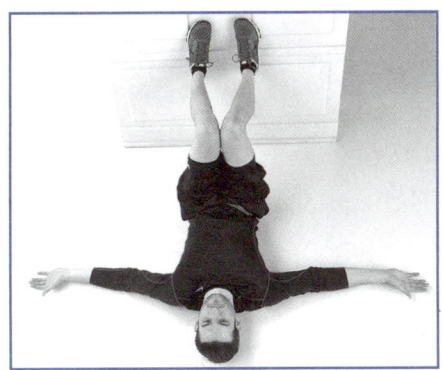
Static Back - Modifications D

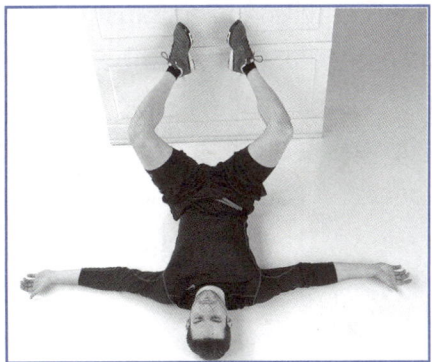
Static Back - Modifications D

Power Over Pain Intelligent Fitness for the Amateur and Professional

■ Exercise – Static Back Pullbacks

(Adapted from Egoscue Method, 2001-2003)

Purpose: This exercise is designed to decrease rotation; properly and bilaterally engage muscles of the hips, low back, quads, and muscles of the lower legs and feet; activate the kinetic chain from the feet to the hips; and reduce low back and hamstring tightness. It decreases compensatory patterns of the hip and torso.

Equipment: Access to a wall or chair, yoga block, small ball (eight to ten inch diameter)

Contraindications/Precautions: None

Process:

1. Assess the discomfort and tightness in your neck, shoulders, torso, low back, hips, thighs, knees, ankles, and feet. Rate these areas from one to ten with ten being the worst.

2. Lie on your back with your knees bent and feet on the wall so that your feet are parallel and hip joint distance apart. Your knees should be directly above your hip joints, forming two ninety-degree angles at the hips and knees. Your trunk should be centered in relationship to your hips and your head should be centered in relationship to shoulders and torso. Your arms should be out to your sides at approximately a forty-five degree angle with your palms up. If you are going to insert a ball or yoga block between your feet and ankles, now is the time to do so. The block or ball allows you to see your hip instability by noting the movement of the block or ball.

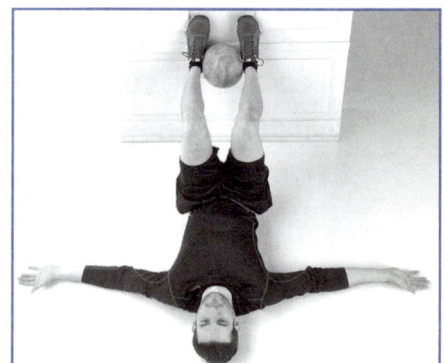

Static Back Pullbacks - Process 2

3. Start this step by taking a slow, deep breath and pull your toes toward your head. Exhale, pulling your lower extremities away from the wall, raising your legs and feet towards the ceiling. Straighten the legs as best as you can so that they are directly above the hip joints. Maintain lower extremities

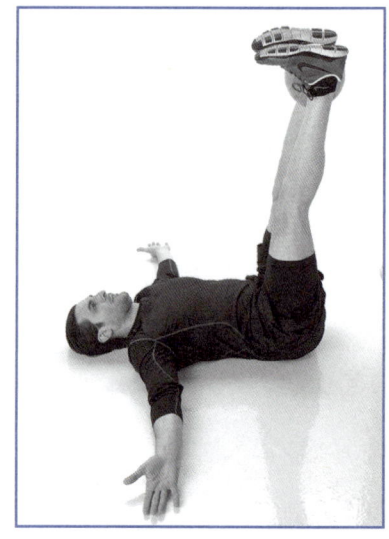

Static Back Pullbacks - Process 3

Section 4: Multi-focal Processes

in this straightened phase for three to five seconds, then return your feet to the original position.

4. Repeat #4 for two minutes. If your hamstrings are tight during this process, concentrate on tightening your quads to reciprocally release your hamstring tightness.

5. Reassess your tightness and discomfort.

■ Exercise – Static Wall

(Adapted from Egoscue, 1998; Egoscue Method, 2001-2003)

Purpose: This exercise is designed to stimulate dynamic tension in the lower extremities and to reduce tightness in the low back, shoulders, and neck. It also helps neutralize the pelvis and reduce torso and hip rotation.

Equipment: Access to a wall

Contraindications/Precautions: None

Process:

1. Assess the discomfort and tightness in your neck, shoulders, torso, low back, hips, thighs, knees, ankles, and feet. Rate these areas from one to ten with ten being the worst.

2. Ideal position: Floor-sit with one side of your body touching a wall and with the arm closest to the wall placed behind your hip. Swing your legs straight up the wall, making sure that the back of your thighs, legs, and heels are touching the wall as you rotate your torso

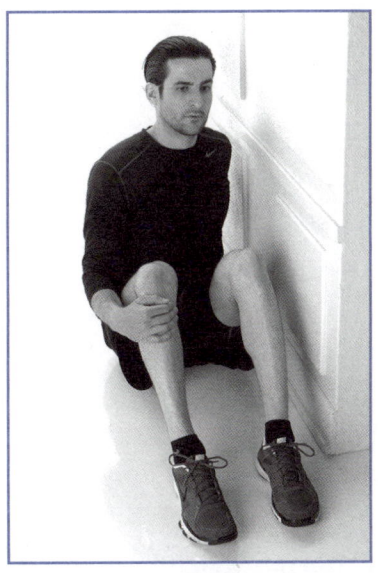
Static Wall - Process 2

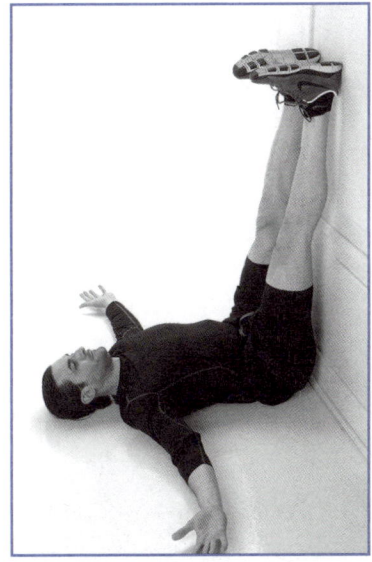
Static Wall - Process 2

onto the floor. If you have tight hamstrings, your hips may need to be further away from the wall but your legs still need to be straight from the hips to the feet. Your toes need to be pulled down toward your face, your feet parallel and inline with the hip joints. Your torso should be perpendicular to the wall and aligned with the hips, and the head should be centered on the body midline. Your arms should be out to the sides of your torso with palms up.

3. Maintain your feet on the wall five minutes, allowing your hips and torso to settle and your hamstrings and gastrocs to relax. A way to expedite hamstring lengthening is by doing quad contractions while in Static Wall position.

4. Reassess the tightness and discomfort in your neck, shoulders, torso, low back, hips, thighs, knees, ankles, and feet.

Modifications:

A. Static Wall with Reverse Presses: After assuming the position of basic Static Wall described in #2 above, place your arms in an upright goalpost position. Press elbows and upper arms, and muscles between the shoulders into the floor, making sure the shoulder joint goes backward and close to the floor. Repeat for two minutes. This process can also be done using **Walking Arm and Shoulder Presses**, page 124.

B. Static Wall with Pullovers: After assuming the position of basic Static Wall described in #2 above, extend your arms above your chest. Keeping your arms close enough so that your thumbs can touch, lower your arms over your head. Limit your range of motion to what you can do with your arms straight. Repeat for two minutes.

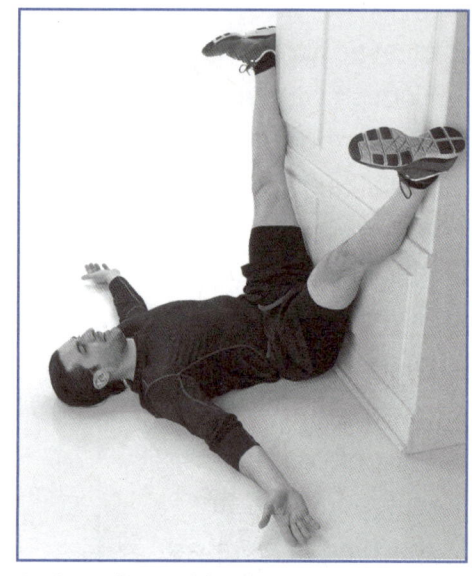

Static Wall - Modification C

C. Static Wall Splits: After assuming the position of basic Static Wall described in #2 above, stay in Static Wall for at least two to three minutes. Keeping the legs against the wall, quads tight and the feet dorsi-flexed,

Section 4: Multi-focal Processes

open your legs without rotating them. Your big toe should face your shoulder and not the floor. Hold this position for at least two to three minutes or until tightness decreases and the hips settle.

D. Static Wall Single Leg Abduction and Hip Stabilization with VersaCuff: Place the VersaCuff around your ankles. Assume the position of basic Static Wall listed in #2 above. Stabilize the left hip and leg (keep them still). Drop the right leg open, keeping the heel on the wall to Static Wall Splits position (Modification C above). Return the right leg to the starting position. Repeat for two minutes. Then stabilize the right hip and leg and open the left leg to Static Wall Splits position. Return the left leg to the starting position. Repeat for two minutes. When opening either leg to the side, be aware of any movement in the stabilizing hip and/or torso. With more repetitions, that movement should diminish.

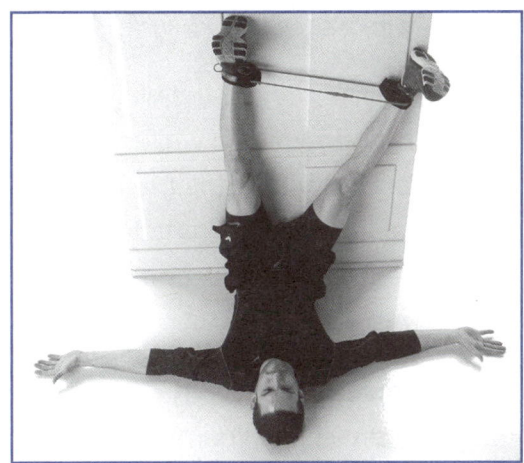

Static Wall - Modification D

■ Exercise – Static Wall Flexion

Purpose: This exercise is designed to increase flexion of the lumbar spine and lower extremities and stretch the muscles of the posterior surface of the body.

Equipment: Access to a wall

Contraindications/Precautions: Since the flexed position mandates that your thighs be close to your abdomen, you might experience pressure, discomfort, or esophageal reflux. If you have a hiatal hernia or excess fat over your abdomen, move your hips out from the wall far enough to relieve the pressure.

Process:

1. Assess the discomfort and tightness in your neck, shoulders, torso, low back, hips, thighs, knees, ankles, and feet. Rate these areas from one to ten with ten being the worst.

2. Ideal position: Floor-sit with one side of your body touching a wall. Swing your legs straight up the wall, making sure that the back of your thighs, legs, and heels are touching the wall. If you have tight hamstrings, your hips may need to be further away from the wall, but your legs still need to be straight from the hips to the feet. Your feet need to be dorsi-flexed, parallel and inline with the hip joints; the torso should be perpendicular to the wall and aligned with the hips; and the head should be centered on the body midline. Your arms should be out to the sides of your torso with palms up.

3. Keeping your feet on the wall, slide them downward while simultaneously bending the knees and maintaining knee and foot alignment with the sits bones.

4. Maintain this flexed position three to five minutes; however, if your muscles are still stretching, you may want to remain in this position longer.

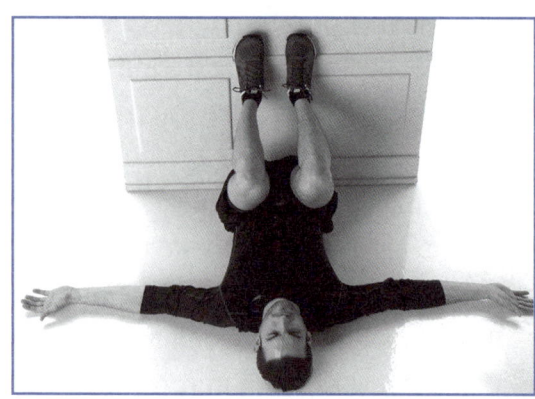

Static Wall Flexion - Process 3

5. Reassess your tightness and discomfort.

■ Exercise – Superman Sequence

Purpose: This process is designed to promote postural alignment and stability of the spine and core. It engages the totality of the posterior kinetic chain so that each body region pulls into extension. Superman helps reduce a rounded back and engages the hips into a more neutral position. The Superman sequence balances each region of the skeleton, front to back and right side to left side. If you have difficulty performing the Superman process or the modifications, see modification E below. This adaptation can be used for any exercise in the Superman Sequence.

Equpment: Small medicine ball, light dumbbells, Thera-Band resistance tubing, VersaCuff

Contraindications/Precautions: If you have bulging discs, most medical sources discourage any hyperextension of the back. If this is your diagnosis, limit your trunk range of motion to neutral rather than trunk hyperextension.

Section 4: Multi-focal Processes

Process:

1. Stand and observe your alignment in a mirror, especially noting if you have any rotation or asymmetry in your trunk, i.e., one shoulder higher than the other or torso not centered over hips. Is your weight distributed equally over both feet and even from heels to toes?

2. Lie face down with your legs and feet pulled to midline and your arms extended above your shoulders.

3. *Without rotating your hips and torso*, lift your right arm up from the floor as far as your body will allow. Hold three to five seconds and breathe. Return right arm to the floor.

   Without rotating your hips and torso, lift your left arm up from the floor as far as your body will allow. Hold three to five seconds and breathe. Return left arm to the floor.

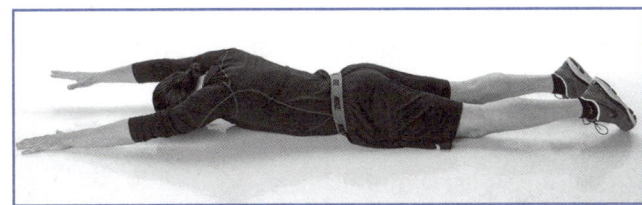

Superman Sequence - Process 3

4. Repeat #3 several times before lifting both arms and head from the floor. Maintain this position for three to five seconds, continuing to breathe.

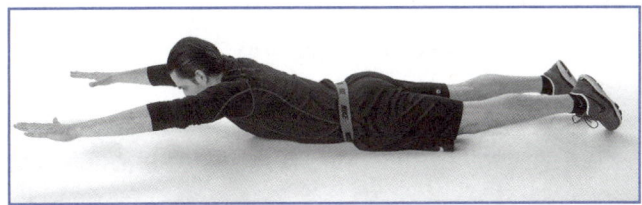

Superman Sequence - Process 4

5. *Without rotating your torso*, lift your right leg up from the floor as far as your hips will allow. Make sure, as you lift your leg from the ground, that the foot stays in line with your hip. Breathe and maintain the position for three to five seconds.

6. Without rotating your hips and torso, lift your left leg up from the floor as far as your hips will allow. Breathe and maintain the position for three to five seconds, keeping your left foot in line with your hip.

7. Repeat #5 and #6 several times before lifting both legs

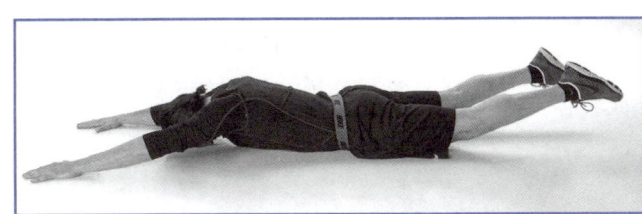

Superman Sequence - Process 7

simultaneously as far as your hips will allow. Maintain the position for three to five seconds and breathe.

8. Alternate lifting both arms and torso with lifting both legs and hips. *Without rotating your hips and torso*, lift right arm and left leg. Maintain this position for three to five seconds and breathe. Lift left arm and right leg and maintain this position for three to five seconds.

9. Lift head, arms, and legs up from the floor and maintain the position while breathing three to five seconds.

Modifications:

A. Superman Starfish: Lift your head and both arms and legs off of the floor. Open them out to your sides. Maintain this open position for three to five seconds and breathe. Return arms and legs to midline and drop them back to the floor.

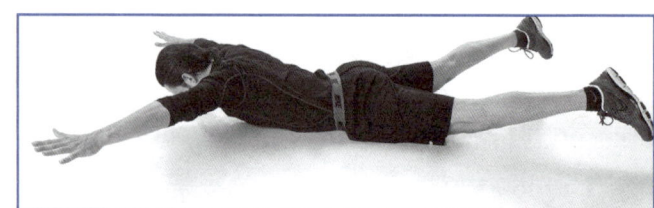

Superman Sequence - Modification A

Note: This can be done using resistance bands around wrists and/or ankles. You can also hold small dumbbells. Repeat this sequence several times. Starfish can be done unilaterally or bilaterally.

B. Superman Rows: Holding small dumbbells, lift your arms and legs up from the floor, keeping them close to midline. Then bending your elbows, bring your arms toward your torso, maintaining this position

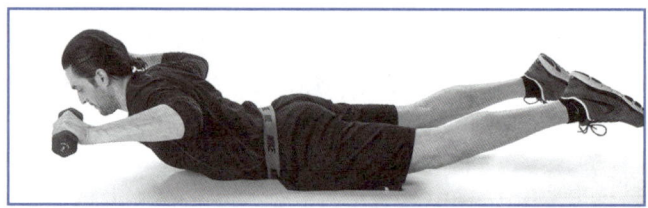

Superman Sequence - Modification B

three to five seconds. Return your arms back to midline, making sure your arms are straight. Drop arms and legs to the ground. Repeat this sequence several times.

Section 4: Multi-focal Processes

C. Superman with Arms to the Side at Shoulder Level: In prone, move your arms out to the side at shoulder level. Lift your head, arms, and legs off of the floor. Breathe and maintain this position for three to five seconds.

Note: This exercise can be done bilaterally with small dumbbells or a resistance tube; it can also be done one arm at a time for increased emphasis on stabilization of the torso and hips.

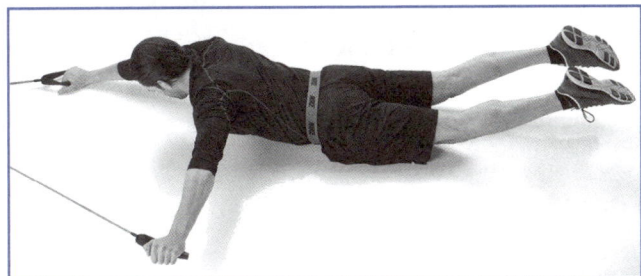

Superman Sequence - Modification C Note

D. Superman with Arms to Small of the Back:

In prone, start with your arms extended above your shoulders and pulled to midline as in #2 above. While focusing on the muscles in your upper and midback, pull your arms toward the small of your back. Keep your elbows straight. Return your arms back to original position and repeat process.

Note: This can be done unilaterally, bilaterally, or alternating your arms and passing a small ball or dumbbell.

E. Superman Postural Adaptation: If you experience any pain or discomfort in the torso or hips during any of the Superman exercises, while in prone, pad your belly to diminish lumbar strain. A towel roll or small ball, three to five inches in diameter placed under your forehead will help protect your cervical curve and provide stabilization. Placing a small ball on your lumbar spine gives you feedback that you are staying still and stable. Should you rotate or shift your hips side to side, the ball will roll off or move.

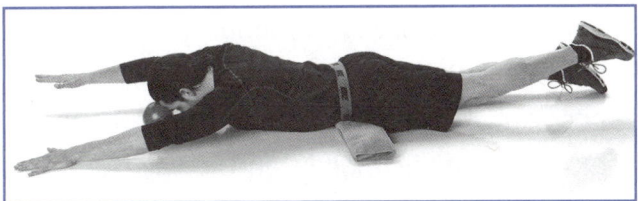

Superman Sequence - Modification E

■ Exercise – Triangle

Purpose: The purpose of this exercise is to promote hip neutrality and stabilization. Triangle influences all load-bearing joints and body regions directly or indirectly. This exercise is one of the most demanding in the manual when done correctly; however, it is one of the most effective in reducing a variety of misalignment pains and discomfort throughout the body.

Equipment: Access to a wall

Contraindications/Precautions: If you have had recent knee or hip surgery, consult your physician.

Process:

1. Assess the tightness, restriction, discomfort, and/or pain that you feel anywhere from feet to head. Rate each area from one to ten with ten being the worst.

2. Stand with your back to a wall with both heels against that surface and feet parallel to each other.

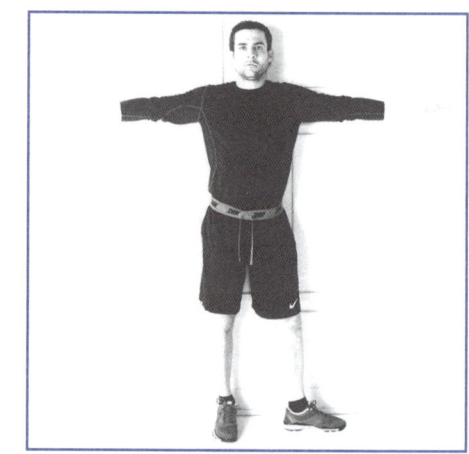

Triangle - Process 4

3. Keep your right foot in place and move the left foot so that it is approximately three inches away from and parallel to the wall. Ideally, the heel of your left foot should be twelve to fourteen inches away from the arch of your right foot.

4. Open your arms at shoulder level. Your head, both hips, and shoulders should be touching the wall. If you cannot maintain your left foot position while your body is touching the wall, move it an additional distance away from the wall while keeping it parallel.

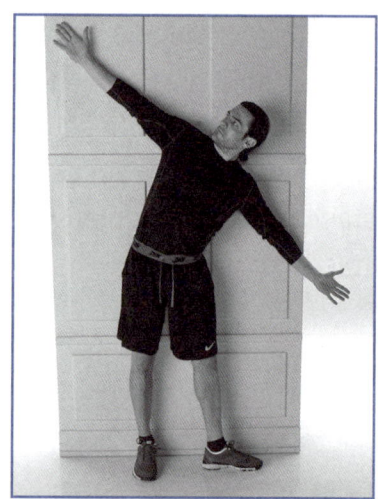

Triangle - Process 5

5. Look at your right hand and lean your torso and left arm to the left toward the floor. Remember your head, shoulders, and hips should all be against the wall.

Section 4: Multi-focal Processes

6. Hold this position for at least one minute, making sure you are breathing deeply. You may experience a constant discomfort anywhere in your body but specifically at your knees and hips. This torque or pull is part of the nature of the repositioning process and should decrease once you have completed the process.

7. Repeat the same process on the other body side.

8. Reassess the tightness, restriction, and/or pain that you noted before you began this process.

■ Exercise – Wall Presses
   (Adapted from Egoscue Method, 2001-2003)

Purpose: This process is designed to reduce rotation and change the dynamic tension of the torso. It also addresses weight distribution and alignment. As you change alignment and weight distribution, you increase the vertical loading component of the entire spine and load-bearing joints.

Equipment: Access to a wall

Contraindications/Precautions: None

Process:

1. Assess the discomfort and tightness in your neck, shoulders, torso, low back, hips, thighs, knees, ankles, and feet. Rate these areas from one to ten with ten being the worst.

2. Stand against the wall with your heels touching it, feet parallel and hip joint distance apart, arms at a forty-five degree angle, palms open with backs of your hands on the wall. The back of your head should be on the wall and centered on the top of the torso.

3. Keeping weight in your heels, press your shoulder blades into the wall and then release. Your sternum should come upward and forward as you press. Hold each repetition three to five seconds.

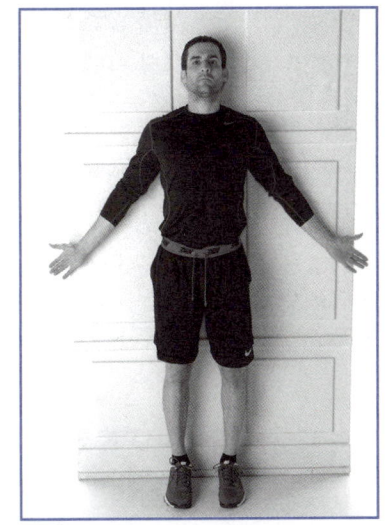

Wall Presses - Process 2

Power Over Pain Intelligent Fitness for the Amateur and Professional

4. Repeat at least fifteen to twenty times.

5. Keeping your shoulders on the wall, drop your chin to your chest. Hold your head in this position and continue to press your shoulder blades into the wall at least fifteen to twenty times.

6. Return your head to upright with the back of the head touching the wall. Turn your hands so that the palms are now touching the wall with your arms straight and at a forty-five degree angle. Continue to press your shoulder blades into the wall at least fifteen to twenty times.

7. Drop your chin to your chest, keeping your palms and the backs of your shoulders on the wall. Continue to press your shoulder blades into the wall at least fifteen to twenty times.

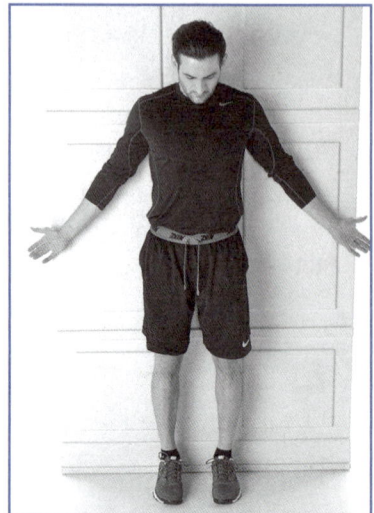

Wall Presses - Process 5

8. Step away from the wall and reassess your tightness and discomfort.

▪ Exercise – Wall Sit

Purpose: This process is for anyone with head, neck, shoulder, torso, low back, hip, knee, ankle, or foot pain or weakness. It serves to reeducate and align major load-bearing joints.

Equipment: Access to a wall, yoga block, strap or pilates ring

Contraindications/Precautions: If you have weak legs or begin to feel discomfort in your knees or thighs, lessen the angle at your hips and knees by sliding your hips upward on the wall. Continue to hold the position.

Process:

1. Stand up and assess your posture noting such things as: vertical alignment, position of your shoulders, trunk and hip rotation, forward weight bearing (weight more in the toes and balls of feet versus weight in the heels), and weight evenly distributed.

Section 4: Multi-focal Processes

2. Start by leaning against a wall and then walk your feet forward about two feet. Your knees should be behind your toes and your feet should be about eight inches apart, toes facing straight ahead, and weight in the heels.

3. Make sure your torso is centered over your hips and your low back; shoulder blades and head are on the wall.

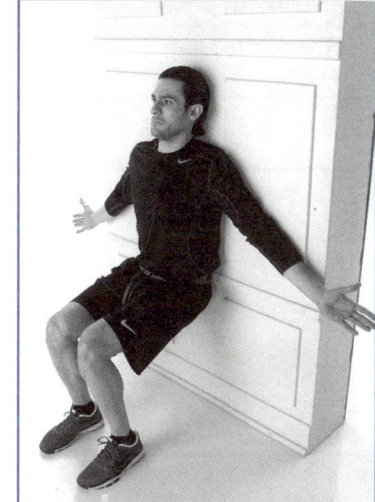

Wall Sit - Process 4

4. Drop your hips downward on the wall so that your knees are bent at approximately ninety degrees or at a level that you can sustain for several seconds, working up to two minutes. If your legs start to fatigue, rather than terminating the exercise, try sliding your hips upwards a few inches and continue to hold the position.

5. Reassess your posture and weight distribution.

Modifications:

A. If your knees and thighs start falling outward, place a yoga block between your knees and hold the block during the process.

B. If your knees and thighs start falling inward, place a yoga strap or Pilates ring above the knees, pushing outward during the process.

Power Over Pain Intelligent Fitness for the Amateur and Professional

My Progress Journal

Exercise Name	Date	Notes

Reward yourself for changing your routine!

Section 5: Respiration

Introduction: Effective respiration is essential for all function and movement; therefore, we felt it is important to give respiration its own section. Take a deep breath! When you inhale fully, the ribcage and diaphragm expand in several dimensions. If you do not see your lower ribcage moving when you inhale, you are not breathing from your diaphragm or maximizing your oxygen capacity. Shallow breathing moves primarily the upper ribcage, collarbones, and neck muscles, promoting a rounded upper back and forward head. Remember, if you hold your breath when exercising, you may elevate your blood pressure. It is important to be aware of how you are breathing.

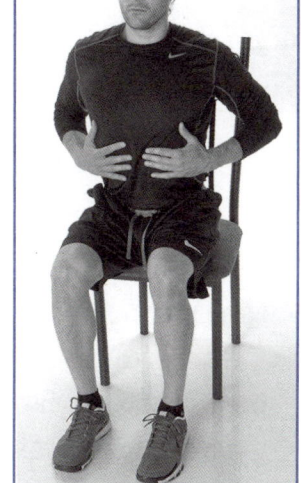

Upward outward chest expansion

■ Exercise – Fragmented Breathing
(Alon, 2007)

Purpose: This exercise is designed to increase your capacity to inhale and exhale deeply.

Equipment: None

Contraindications/Precautions: None

Process:

1. Assessment: Lie in supine with bent knees. This is a two-step assessment.

A. Assess any tightness and restriction of your ribcage and diaphragm by pressing along the ribs on both left and right body sides from armpit to above the waist. Is there any give or spring to the ribs, or do they feel rigid and tight?

Power Over Pain Intelligent Fitness for the Amateur and Professional

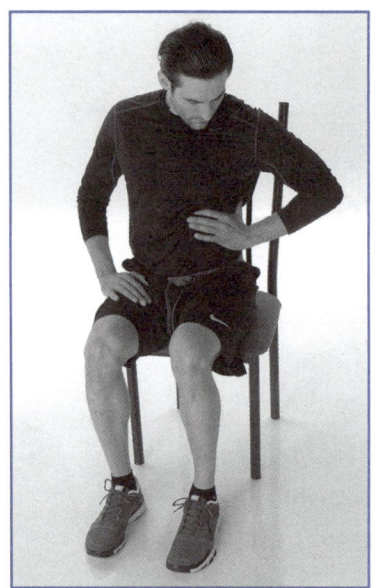

Assess rib spring - Process 1A

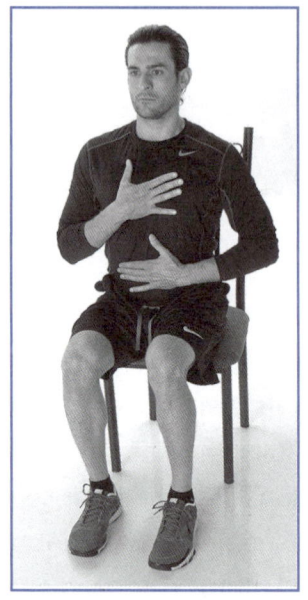

Fragmented Breathing - Process 1B

B. Now place one hand over your sternum and your other hand so that you can feel the action of your diaphragm (about four inches above your navel). Take a deep breath, noting which hand moves upward. Ideally, it should be the hand over your diaphragm. All breaths should be taken in through the nose and exhaled out the mouth.

2. Take a deep breath, inhaling through your nose. Open your mouth and exhale in continuous short spurts, using the syllable HA as many times as you can until the exhalation is complete. This constitutes one cycle of fragmented exhalation.

3. Repeat #2 at least three times.

4. Now inhale through the nose in continuous short spurts as many times as you times as you can until the inhalation is complete, then exhale normally through your mouth. This constitutes one fragmented inhalation cycle.

5. Repeat #4 at least three times.

Section 5: Respiration

■ Exercise - VersaStep Breathing

Purpose: This exercise is designed to decrease the restriction in the diaphragm and ribcage, ultimately improving respiration.

Equipment: VersaStep, yoga block or small pillow

Contraindications/Precautions: None

Process:

1. While remaining in supine with bent knees, center a VersaStep at the base of your ribcage, textured side up, and a yoga block or small pillow under your head. Your arms should be positioned at shoulder level with palms up and hands open. Feet should be parallel and aligned with sits bones.

2. Keeping your hips, legs, and feet fairly still, slowly shift your torso to the right over the VersaStep while your shoulders remain back towards the floor. Now return your ribcage to center and take a deep breath. Move your torso slowly to the left over the VersaStep, remembering to keep your shoulders back towards the floor and take another breath. This is one cycle.

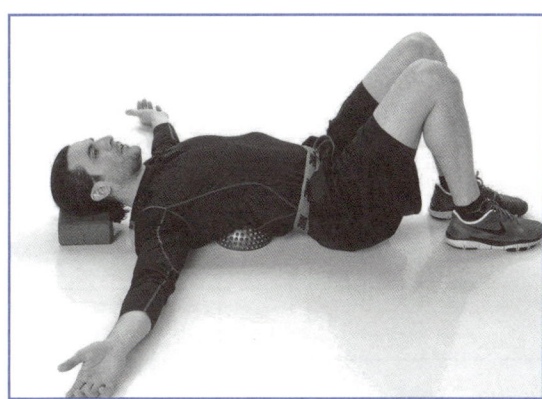
VersaStep Breathing - Process 2

3. Repeat for at least five cycles.

4. Reassess the amount of tightness and restriction in your ribcage and diaphragm by repeating A, B, and C listed in Fragmented Breathing above.

Note: There are two processes in other sections of the book (Standing Windmill in the Section 4: Multi-focal and Double Leg Drop with Mini-windmills in Section 12 Upper Thoracic/ Processes) that enhance respiration because they eliminate tightness around the ribcage.

Power Over Pain Intelligent Fitness for the Amateur and Professional

My Progress Journal		
Exercise Name	**Date**	**Notes**

Tomorrow is now!

Section 6: The Power of Postural Alignment

Introduction: Human posture is the dynamic interrelationship of body parts to one another. When standing, all body regions should be stacked symmetrically one over another like a pillar. Proper alignment produces optimal load-bearing capability and allows the body to withstand gravity.

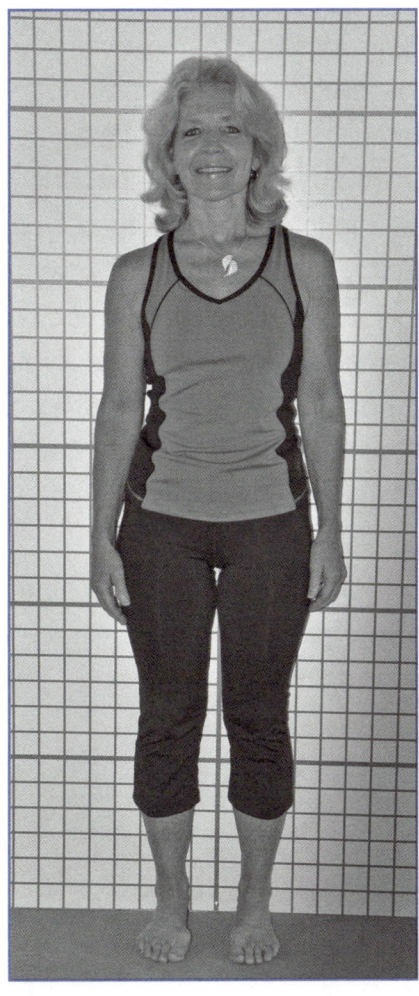
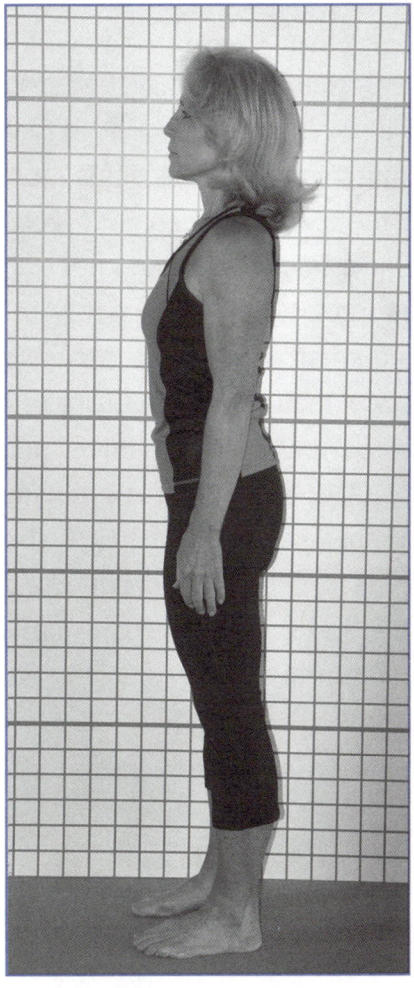

Your postural alignment is a direct reflection of what you do most of the time. We call this **occupationally induced posture**. If you sit at your computer all day and are sedentary in general, you are more likely to have a rounded thoracic back and forward head and shoulders. Alternatively, if you are active and make the effort to do the exercises in this book, you will have improved alignment and produce increased quality of movement. There is also a direct relationship between your postural alignment, fatigue, soft tissue strain, injury, and pain. The better you are aligned, the less fatigue, strain, or injury you will have. The better your muscles are balanced, the less pain you will experience.

With ideal postural alignment, you will be more successful withstanding a test to your balance. In other words, you will be more stable with good posture and able to navigate over uneven terrain or sustain balance even when suddenly challenged. Aligned trunk and pelvis improves head and neck position and all extremity function. Profound positive effects occur to all body systems by correctly positioning body regions. For example, the digestive system works more efficiently in a person with good posture versus someone with faulty posture.

Your musculoskeletal system is more secure with proper alignment. While standing, the space between your feet should be hip joint distance apart, your feet aligned under your knees and knees under your hip joints. This establishes a good **base of support (BOS)** on which to stand. When you stand with your feet close to midline, you narrow your BOS, increasing the demand for core strength. While standing with feet wider than hip joint distance does increase your BOS, it produces stress at the knees, feet, and ankles and conversely decreases stability. Your **center of gravity (COG)** is the point about which your weight is evenly distributed. When you are properly aligned, your COG should be directly over your BOS.

There is no shortcut to producing good postural alignment. It takes time, persistence, and specific exercises that address your particular postural issues. The following postural checklist will help you assess and determine appropriate exercises for your needs.

Section 6: The Power of Postural Alignment

Postural Alignment Checklist

Feet/Ankles	Yes	No
Are your feet parallel to each other?		
Is one foot or are both feet turned in?		
Is one foot or are both feet turned out?		
Is one foot farther forward than the other? If so, which foot?		
Is your weight equally distributed on both feet?		
Is your weight in your heels or on the balls of your feet?		
Are your feet/ankles pronated?		
Are your feet/ankles supinated?		

Knees	Yes	No	Right	Left
Do your feet align under your knees?				
Do your kneecaps face forward?				
Do your kneecaps face inward?				
Do your kneecaps face outward?				
Are your kneecaps tilted?				
Is one kneecap higher than the other?				
Do your knees align under your hips?				
In side view, is your knee joint lined up over your ankle?				
Are your knee joints forward of your ankles?				
Are your knee joints behind your ankles?				

Postural Alignment Checklist

Hips/Trunk	Yes	No	Right	Left
Which description most resembles your hips?				
Anterior tipped				
Neutral position				
Posterior tipped				
Right hip forward (counterclockwise rotation)				
Left hip forward (clockwise rotation)				
Do you have lordosis?				
Do you have kyphosis?				
Do you have lateral flexion? If so, which side?				
Is your trunk rotated?				
Are your hips in flexion?				
Is your trunk in flexion?				
Are your hips hyperextended?				
Is your trunk hyperextended?				
Is your trunk centered over your hips?				

Section 6: The Power of Postural Alignment

Postural Alignment Checklist

Shoulders	Yes	No	Right	Left
Are your shoulders level?				
If not, which one is higher?				
Are your shoulders positioned directly above your hips?				
Are your shoulders positioned forward of hips?				
Are your shoulders positioned behind the hips?				
Are your shoulder blades flat on your back?				
Do your shoulder blades protrude?				
Which of the following descriptors below best describes the relationship of the top of the scapula to your shoulder?				
At the same level as the shoulder?				
Higher than the top of the shoulder?				
Lower than the top surface of the shoulder?				
When standing relaxed, do your hands/arms hang:				
At your side?				
In front of your hips?				
Behind your hips?				
Which of the following describes your hand position?				
Back of your hand facing forward?				
Thumb forward?				
Palm forward?				

Postural Alignment Checklist

Neck/Head	Yes	No	Right	Left
Is your head centered over your midline?				
In side view, is the back of your ear lined up with the shoulder hip, knee, and ankle joints?				
Is your head tilted right or left?				
Is your head rotated clockwise?				
Is your head rotated counterclockwise?				
Do you have a cervical curve?				
Is your neck strained in any way?				

Common Types of Postural Maladaptations and Exercise Recommendations

Postural Pattern 1: Forward head, forward shoulders, rounded thoracic back with posterior pelvic tilt

    A. Sternum Tilts (Section 12: Upper Thoracic/Shoulder Processes) page 122.

    B. Walking Arm and Shoulder Presses (Shoulder Arm Glide Progression Section 12: Upper Thoracic/Shoulder Processes) page 124.

    C. Cats and Dogs (Section 4: Multi-focal Processes) page 16.

    D. Sitting Floor Elbow Curls (Section 4: Multi-focal Processes) page 31.

    E. Arm Circles (Section 4: Multi-focal Processes) page 15.

    F. Superman Sequence (Section 4: Multi-focal Processes) page 44.

Section 6: The Power of Postural Alignment

Postural Pattern 2: Asymmetrical posture with one shoulder and/or one hip higher than the other

    A. Gravity Drop (Section 4: Multi-focal Processes) page 21.

    B. Standing Windmill (Section 4: Multi-focal Processes) page 35.

    C. Static Wall with Pullovers (Section 4: Multi-focal Processes) page 42.

    D. Double Leg Drop with Mini-windmills (Section 12: Upper Thoracic/Shoulder Processes) page 116.

    E. Bilateral Horizontal Roll (Section 10: Hip/Low Back Stability Processes) page 96.

Postural Pattern 3: Head forward, upper back and neck strain, Increased lordotic curve, sagging gut

    A. Static Wall with Pullovers (Section 4: Multi-focal Processes) page 42.

    B. Prone Ankle Squeezes (Section 4: Multi-focal Processes) page 27.

    C. Wall Presses (Section 4: Multi-focal Processes) page 49.

    D. Wall Sit (Section 4: Multi-focal Processes) page 50.

    E. Static Back Pullbacks (Section 4: Multi-focal Processes) page 40.

Postural Pattern 4: Anterior pelvic tilt, hyperextended knees, everted feet

    A. Frog (Section 4: Multi-focal Processes) page 19.

    B. Prone Ankle Squeezes (Section 4: Multi-focal Processes) page 27.

    C. Wall Sit (Section 4: Multi-focal Processes) page 50.

    D. Sit-to-stand (Section 4: Multi-focal Processes) page 28.

    E. Inline Gluteal Contractions (Section 4: Multi-focal Processes) page 25.

Postural Pattern 5: Decreased lumbar curve with posterior pelvic tilt, flexed knees, everted feet

A. Pelvic Tilts Using the VersaStep (Section 10: Hip/Low Back Stability Processes) page 103.

B. Bridging (Section 10: Hip/Low Back Stability Processes) page 98.

C. Medial and Lateral Hip Stabilization (Section 10: Hip/Low Back Stability Processes) page 101.

D. Triangle (Section 10: Hip/Low Back Stability Processes) page 48.

Postural Pattern 6: Posterior pelvic tilt with hyperextended knees

A. Prone Ankle Squeezes (Section 4: Multi-focal Processes) page 27.

B. Pelvic Tilts Using the VersaStep (Section 10: Hip/Low Back Stability Processes) page 103.

C. Cats and Dogs (Section 4: Multi-focal Processes) page 16.

D. Superman Sequence (Section 4: Multi-focal Processes) page 44.

Section 6: The Power of Postural Alignment

My Progress Journal

Exercise Name	Date	Notes

You are in charge of your progress!

Section 7: Restoring or Improving Balance

Introduction: Balance is defined as stability of body or mind equilibrium. In addition to this section, many of the processes in other areas of the book will also help develop or restore balance. Assuming your central nervous system's balance mechanisms are functioning normally, additional factors for good balance include: postural alignment, proper joint loading, muscular balance, and hip stability. One additional concept essential to understanding balance is the center of gravity defined as the equilibrium point in a balanced or supported body where all its weight is concentrated.

If you are standing in good postural alignment, your feet are parallel to each other and are directly under your hip joints. This arrangement of feet to hips creates an ideal base of support and efficient joint loading of the lower extremities. The quality of your base of support is directly related to your balance. If your feet are too close together, your base of support is too narrow to promote ideal balance in sustained standing. If your feet are too wide apart, you also reduce the quality of your base of support since the femurs are not directly under the pelvis. An additional element for ideal balance is that your center of gravity should be directly over your base of support.

When you develop your sense of balance through training, challenges to your equilibrium result in automatic musculoskeletal adjustments. Understand that in order to improve and train your balance, it will be necessary to be out of balance. For this reason, we recommend having a partner to spot or assist you in the beginning.

Once you start to improve your balance secondarily to improvements in postural alignment, you may experience transient dizziness as you move from one posture to another.

For example, if you are working on realignment in a supine position and transition to upright, you might notice some dizziness for a few seconds. This is a normal response as part of your balance restoration. In this scenario, make sure you position your feet for the ideal base of support.

Power Over Pain Intelligent Fitness for the Amateur and Professional

Note: Exercises in this section are listed according to difficulty from simple to more challenging and are not arranged alphabetically. Arm patterns in a variety of movement planes can be added to the BOSU or ball exercises in order to increase the balance challenge.

■ Exercise – Kneeling on a BOSU

Purpose: This process is designed to assist you in responding adaptively to a balance challenge on an unstable surface.

Equipment: A BOSU

Note: a balance disc may be substituted for a BOSU

Contraindications/Precautions: If you have Meniere's disease or any other type of dizziness, do not do this process alone.

Process:

1. Place the BOSU on the floor on its flat side. Assess your ability to kneel on the BOSU. Are you making huge adjustments with your arms and trunk? Do you need to touch your toes on the floor? Rate your efficiency in maintaining your balance from one to ten with ten attributed to many compensatory movements and constant re-adjustment.

2. Now adjust your knees and thighs so that they are parallel and equidistance from the center of the BOSU keeping your toes up off the floor, if you can.

3. Place your arms out to the side at shoulder height making sure you engage your abdominal muscles and the muscles between your shoulder blades. Lift and lower your arms bilaterally twelve to fifteen times. Then try lifting and lowering your left arm twelve to fifteen times with your right arm at your side. Switch to lifting and lowering your right arm twelve to fifteen times with your left arm at your side.

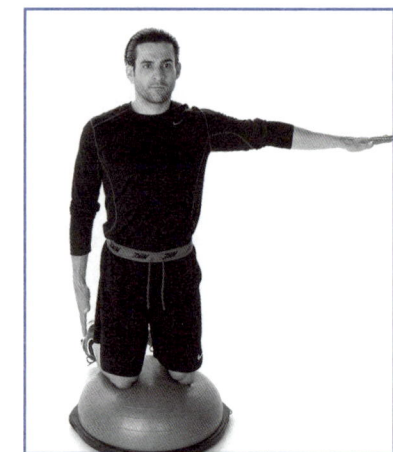

Kneeling on a BOSU - Process 3

4. Attempt to lift and lower both arms up above your head twelve to fifteen times, palms facing each other. Now, keep your right arm at your side and lift and lower your left arm above your head. Repeat twelve to fifteen times. Switch to lifting and lowering your right arm with your left arm at your side. Repeat twelve to fifteen times.

5. Raise your right arm above your head and your left arm to the side at shoulder height. Switch to your left arm above your head and your right arm to the side at shoulder height. Alternate between the two positions twelve to fifteen times.

6. Reassess your balance.

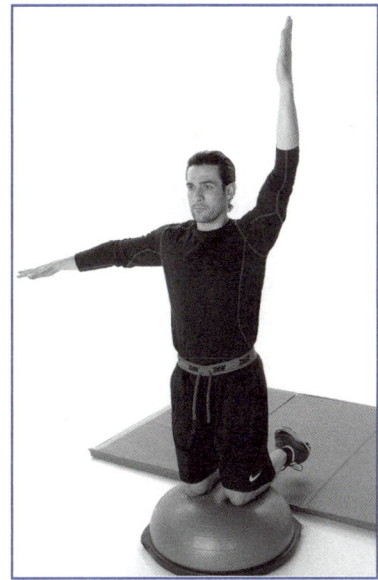
Kneeling on a BOSU - Process 5

Note: You can perform these exercises using small dumbbells. Experiment changing arm pattern such as arm circles or diagonal movements.

■ Exercise – Sitting on a Stability Ball

Purpose: This process is designed to increase awareness of your position in space and your muscle engagement. It also improves confidence in your ability to maintain balance in simple movement.

Equipment: A corner of a room and a stability ball

Contraindications/Precautions: If you have Meniere's disease or any other type of dizziness, do not do this process alone.

Process:

1. Place a stability ball in the corner of a room leaving six inches between the ball and the corner. Sit with your back to the corner, and assess the degree of difficulty you have in keeping your balance and the ball still. Rate the difficulty from one to ten with ten being the most difficult.

2. Sit on the ball with your feet on the floor, so that they are parallel and ideally positioned hip joint distance apart.

3. Experiment with your postural alignment, and see what positions allow you to feel the most comfortable and secure.

4. Practice tilting your pelvis forward and back until these movements are easy.

5. Now move your pelvis right to left until this set of movements is simple. Make sure you are keeping your feet stationary.

6. Now make clockwise circles with your pelvis and upon mastery change to counterclockwise circles.

7. Reassess your ease of balancing on the ball.

Note: There are many other motions you can do on the stability ball. As you become more proficient, you can attempt more complex movements and move the ball out of the corner.

■ Exercise – Standing on a BOSU

Purpose: This exercise enhances your balance responses in standing.

Equipment: A BOSU

Contraindications/Precautions: If you have Meniere's disease or any other type of dizziness, do not do this process alone.

Process:

1. Place the BOSU on the floor on its flat side. Assess your ability to stand on the BOSU. Can you maintain standing on top of the BOSU? Are you making huge adjustments with your arms and trunk? Rate your efficiency in maintaining your balance from one to ten with ten attributed to many compensatory movements and constant readjustment.

2. Now adjust your feet and legs so that they are parallel and equidistance from the center of the BOSU. Your arms should be at your sides.

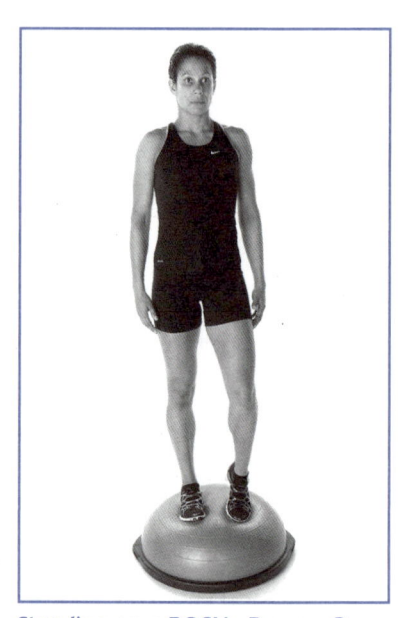

Standing on a BOSU - Process 3

Section 7: Restoring or Improving Balance

3. Keeping your toes in place on the BOSU lift and lower your left heel. Now repeat with the right heel. Repeat fifteen to twenty times. When moving the feet individually becomes simple, progress to lifting and lowering your heels simultaneously as if you are walking in place. Notice if you are shifting and leaning, or if you are able to keep your torso completely still.

4. Add a slight bilateral arm swing (one forward, one back) to the movement in #3.

5. Reassess your ability to stand on the BOSU.

Note: There are numerous modifications that can be made to this sequence, such as marching in place, swinging one leg from front to back, etc.

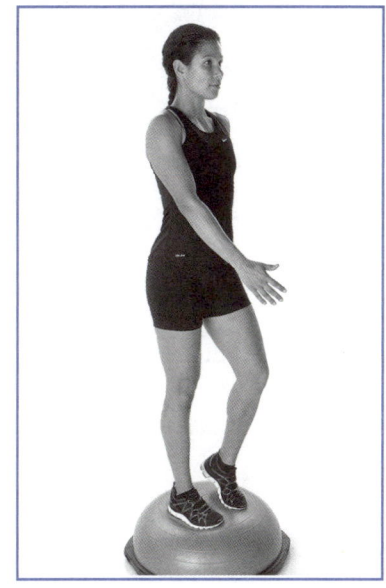

Standing on a BOSU - Process 4

My Progress Journal		
Exercise Name	**Date**	**Notes**

Power Over Pain Intelligent Fitness for the Amateur and Professional

My Progress Journal

Exercise Name	Date	Notes

Slow but sure progress beats no progress!

Section 8: Foot/Ankle Processes

■ Exercise - Alternating Heel Toe

Purpose: You should do Alternating Heel Toe If you are lacking ankle flexibility, have flat arches, or are experiencing pain in feet, ankles, lower legs, or knees. This exercise serves to help develop the longitudinal arch of the foot and reeducate the muscles of the lower leg.

Equipment: None required. For modification of the process, you can use a VersaStep or a small massage ball.

Contraindications/Precautions: If you have diabetic peripheral neuropathy and/or have tenderness in the instep, you will want to either put a towel over the VersaStep or wear padded socks. Padded socks are often found as adaptive equipment for those having diabetic peripheral neuropathy.

Process:

1. Determine the level of flexibility, pain, and range of motion you have in your feet and ankles. Rate them from one to ten with ten being the most rigid and painful.

2. Assume supine bent knee position. Point and flex the right foot and ankle, alternately touching the toes then heel of the right foot to the floor. Try to keep your foot in the same spot throughout the process.

3. Repeat number two with the left foot.

4. Reassess flexibility, pain, and range of motion in your feet and ankles.

Modifications:

A. Alternating Heel Toe on Equipment: You can do alternating heel toe movement over a small foam roller, a VersaStep, or a massage ball.

B. Alternating Heel Toe in Sitting: Sit upright on the edge of a chair or stability ball and position left foot slightly forward. Point and flex the left foot and ankle alternately touching the toes then heel of the left foot to the floor. Repeat number two with the right foot.

C. Alternating Heel Toe in Sitting with Right Ankle Over Left Knee: Sit upright on the edge of a chair or stability ball with knees at ninety degrees flexion and feet on the floor, directly under your knees. Cross your right ankle over your left knee. Align your torso directly over your hips. Point and flex the right foot and ankle making sure to align the left hip directly underneath the left shoulder. While doing this process, you may experience sensation in other joints or areas not directly involved with the movement of the foot/ankle. Alternation of heel/toe can be attempted on the left foot in this position. Repeat this process with the left foot over the right knee.

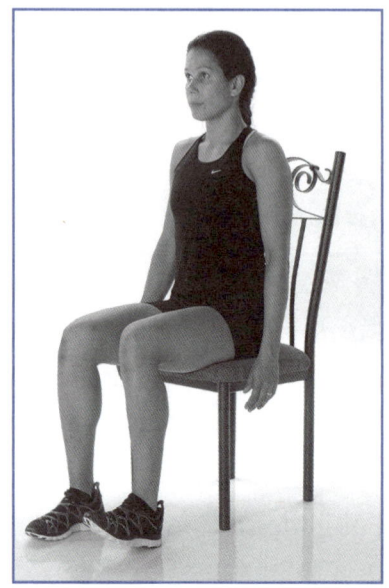

Alternating Heel Toe - Modification B

■ Exercise - Dorsi and Plantar Flexion with a Block in Sitting

Purpose: The purpose of this process is to reeducate muscles of the lower leg when you experience foot and ankle pain. This process can help realign the feet for individuals who toe out in walking or standing.

Equipment: yoga block and a solid, sturdy chair

Contraindication/Precautions: None

Process:

1. Using a scale of one to ten with ten being the worst, assess the amount of foot and ankle pain or discomfort that you have.

2. Remove your shoes and sit on the front edge of the chair. Place a yoga block between your feet, wide side down parallel to the feet. Make sure you are sitting in good postural alignment.

3. Keeping the block between your feet, raise and then lower your toes off the floor. Repeat at least twenty to twenty-five times.

4. Reassess the amount of pain or discomfort in feet or ankles and change in foot position while walking.

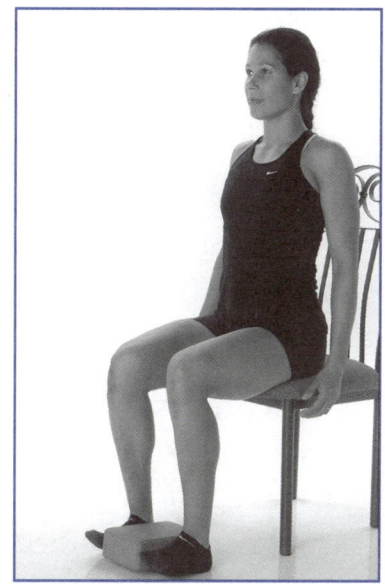

Dorsi and Plantar Flexion with a Block in Sitting - Process 2

■ Exercise - Foot Circles

Purpose: You should do foot circles If you are lacking flexibility and/or stability, have flat arches, or are experiencing pain in feet, ankles, or knees. This exercise serves to increase range of motion and reeducate the muscles and bony alignment of the foot and ankle.

Equipment: Chair or stability ball

Contraindications/Precautions: None

Process:

1. Remove your shoes and determine the level of flexibility, pain, and range of motion you have in your feet and ankles. Rate them from one to ten with ten being the most rigid and painful.

2. Assume supine bent knee position and lift right foot off the ground about three to six inches.

3. Using the right foot, make large, clockwise circles, keeping the lower leg stationary. Repeat thirty times. Make the foot circles as large as you can. It is normal to experience some discomfort as you engage the muscles of foot and ankle.

4. Continue with thirty counterclockwise circles.

5. Return the right foot to the floor, making sure the right heel is aligned with the right sits bone.

6. Repeat the same process clockwise and counterclockwise with the left foot raised, and then rest.

7. Reassess the level of flexibility, pain, and range of motion you have in your feet and ankles.

Modifications:

A. Foot Circles, Knee Extension in Sitting: Sit upright on the edge of a chair or on a stability ball with left leg bent, knee aligned over left foot, right leg extended and slightly elevated from the floor.

Using the right foot, make a large, slow clockwise circle. Repeat thirty times, and then proceed to thirty counterclockwise circles. Return right foot to floor, aligning right knee over right foot, and rest. Repeat the same process with the left foot and ankle, then rest.

B. Foot Circles, Right Ankle over Left Knee in Sitting: Sit upright on the edge of a chair or stability ball with right ankle over left knee. Align your torso directly over your hips. Using the right foot and ankle, make large, slow clockwise circles. Repeat thirty times, and then proceed to thirty counterclockwise circles. Return right foot to floor, aligning right knee over right foot, and rest. Repeat the same process with the left foot and ankle, then rest.

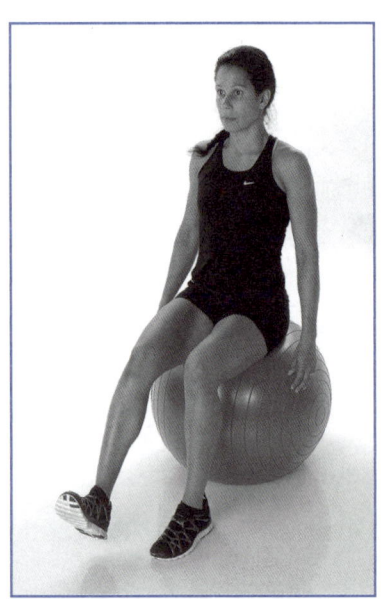

Foot Circles - Modification A

C. Foot Circles Standing: Stand on left foot with right leg positioned slightly forward and elevated from the ground. You may place your left hand on a chair back or stationary object to assist in balance and stability if needed. Using the right foot, make large, clockwise circles. Repeat thirty times. Continue with thirty

Section 8: Foot/Ankle Processes

counterclockwise circles. Return right foot to floor, aligning right foot under right hip, and rest. Repeat the same process clockwise and counterclockwise with the left foot and ankle then rest. Continue with thirty counterclockwise circles. Rest if necessary.

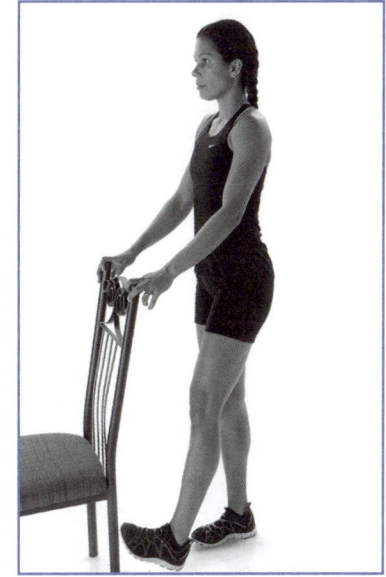
Foot Circles - Modification C

■ Exercise - Heel Cord Lengthening in Supine with a Strap

Purpose: This exercise is designed to lengthen the heel cord and calf muscles.

Equipment: Four-to-five-foot-long strap with buckle or small loop on one end

Contraindications/Precautions: If your heel cords are excessively tight, proceed with caution.

Process:

1. Go into lunge position and assess the tightness of your heel cord, calf, and hamstring muscles on the back leg. Rate the tightness from one to ten with ten being the tightest. Assess both legs.

2. Lie on your back with your left knee bent and left foot on the floor. Make a small loop in your strap and place it around your right foot at the arch. Hold the strap in one or both hands, keeping the back of your shoulders on the floor. Pull your right toes toward your body and straighten your right leg so that you feel a stretch on your

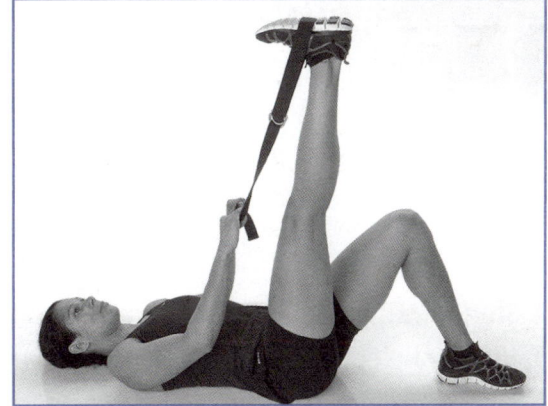
Heel Cord Lengthening in Suprine with a Strap - Process 2

77

heel cords. You may also feel a tug behind your knee or in your hamstrings. Hold this position for at least one minute.

3. Move the strap to the ball of the right foot. Pull your toes toward your body and straighten your right leg. Hold this position for at least one minute.

4. Repeat #2 and #3 on your left foot.

5. Reassess the tightness of your heel cords, calves, and hamstring muscles.

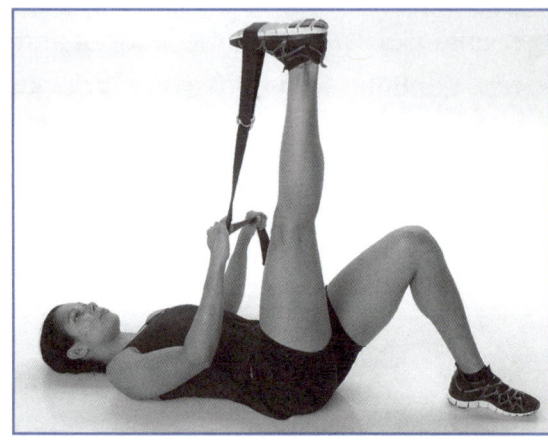

Heel Cord Lengthening in Suprine with a Strap - Process 3

■ Exercise – Heel (Calf) Raises

Purpose: Heel raises are designed to increase the range of motion at the ankle as well as engaging all of the lower leg muscles. It also promotes improved balance.

This process is often called calf raises. It is really the heels that are raised, engaging the calf muscles. We will refer to these exercises as Heel Raises

Equipment: The bottom step of a set of stairs or a step bench or stability ball

Contraindications/Precautions: If you have tight heel cords, proceed slowly and with caution.

Process:

1. Start by assessing pain and range of motion in your feet/ankles from one to ten with ten being the worst.

2. Stand on the edge of a step with the balls of your feet at the edge, heels free. Place one hand on the wall or railing, making sure the body is aligned

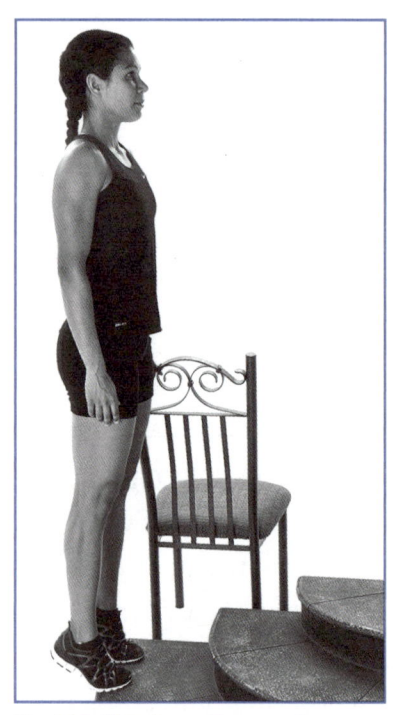

Heel (Calf) Raises - Process 2

Section 8: Foot/Ankle Processes

over the feet. If you need more assistance with balance, make sure you have a railing or chair on both sides of you.

3. Drop both heels below the edge of the step.

4. Raise the heels so that you are on the balls of your feet.

5. Repeat the process from #2, working on full range of motion at the ankle.

6. Reassess pain and range of motion.

Modifications:

A. Heel Raises with a Stability Ball: Facing the wall, place a stability ball against the wall at chest level. While leaning on the ball, place your arms on either side of the ball. Move your feet at least eighteen to twenty inches away from the wall, making sure they are equidistant. Raise your heels so that you are on the balls of your feet, then lower or drop your heels to the floor. Repeat for one to two minutes, gradually increasing your stamina and attempting full range of motion.

B. Unilateral Heel Raises: Both of the above heel raise processes can be done on a single leg by placing one foot on the back of the other heel.

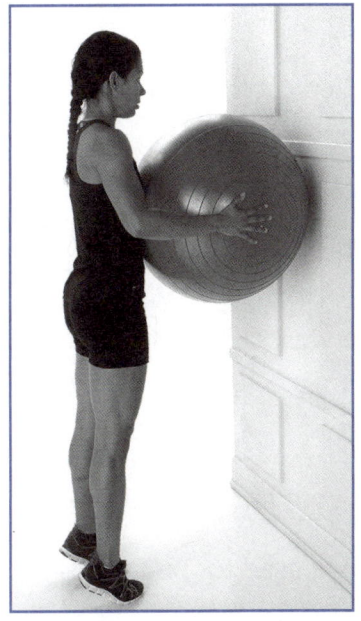
Heel (Calf) Raises - Modification A

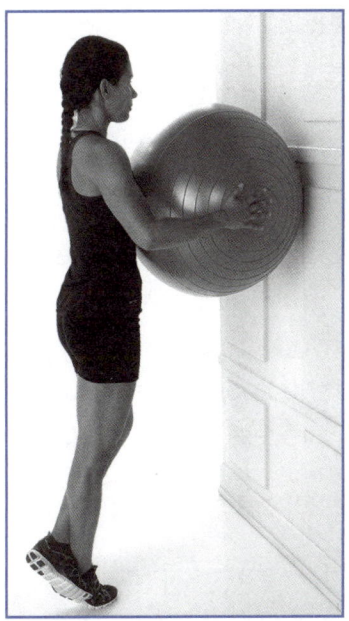
Heel (Calf) Raises - Modification B

Power Over Pain Intelligent Fitness for the Amateur and Professional

■ Exercise - Prehensile Feet and Toe Spreading

Purpose: This process increases the flexibility and mobility of the toes and feet and enhance the gait process.

Equipment: Washcloth, pedicure toe spreaders

Contraindications/Precautions: None

Process:

1. Assess the range of motion in the joints of the toes and feet. Rate flexibility and mobility from one to ten with ten being the tightest and least flexible.

2. Place a washcloth on the floor in front of your right foot. Stand upright in good alignment and attempt to grab the washcloth with the toes of your right foot.

3. If you succeed in picking up the washcloth, release it back to the floor. The act of releasing the cloth extends and separates the toes. Repeat this process twelve to fifteen times.

4. Now do this process with the left foot, following the steps listed in #2 and #3.

5. Place the washcloth on the floor behind your right foot. Extend the right hip back so that you can grab the washcloth with the toes of your right foot. If you succeed in picking up the washcloth, release it to the floor behind you. Repeat this process twelve to fifteen times.

6. Repeat steps one to five with your left foot.

7. Place a toe spreader (as in those used for pedicures) between the toes of both feet. Leave them in place for three to five minutes then remove them.

8. Reassess the range of motion in the joints of your toes and feet.

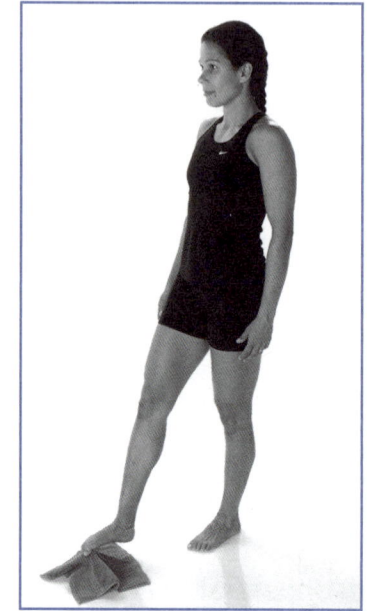

Prehensile Feet an Toe Spreading - Process 2

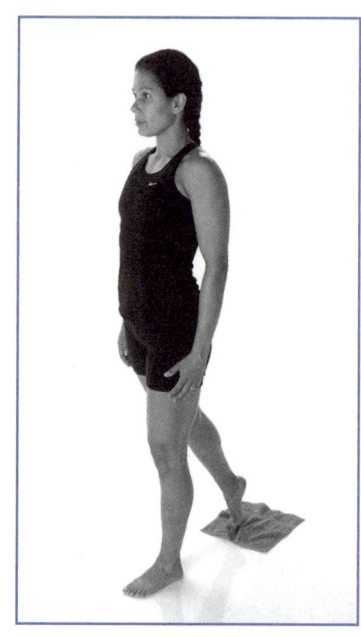

Prehensile Feet an Toe Spreading - Process 5

Section 8: Foot/Ankle Processes

■ Exercise – Toe Raises Leaning on the Wall

Purpose: This exercise strengthens the muscles on the front and outside of the lower leg (anterior tibialis and peroneus muscles) and lengthens the calf muscles (gastronemius and soleus muscles). It is designed to help diminish pain resulting from shin splints.

Equipment: A wall or door

Contraindications/Precautions: None

Process:

1. Rate the pain associated with shin splints from one to ten with ten being the worst.

2. Lean back against a wall or door and walk your feet forward away from the wall eight to ten inches. Your arms should be relaxed at your sides. Feet should be parallel and hip joint distance apart, and your weight should be in your heels.

3. Slowly raise your toes off the floor as far as you can, keeping your feet parallel. Lower your toes back to the floor.

4. Repeat #3, five to six times and build your tolerance to three sets of fifteen to twenty repetitions.

5. Reassess your pain associated with shin splints.

■ Exercise – Wall Drop
   (Adapted from Egoscue, 2001-2003)

Purpose: This exercise lengthens the heel cords, calf, and hamstring muscles. It also changes the distribution of weight into the heels and helps to eliminate rotation.

Equipment: Slant board/wedge.

Contraindications/Precautions: None other than if you are extremely tight, start with the lowest setting on the slant board/wedge.

Process:

1. Stand as you would normally and assess your weight distribution, front of your feet to back, left foot to right foot. Go into lunge position and assess the tightness of

your heel cord, calf, and hamstring muscles on the back leg. Rate the tightness from one to ten with ten being the tightest. Assess both legs.

2. Set the slant board/wedge on a nonslip mat or rug with the narrow end against the wall.

3. Step onto the board with your heels against the wall. Make sure your feet are parallel under your hips. Your back, shoulders, and head should all touch the wall. If your posture does not allow this alignment, do not force your body into the wall.

4. Allow gravity to reposition your vertical alignment over your heels and lengthen tight muscles. Remain in this position for three to five minutes unless you have plantar fasciitis. In this case, remain on the wedge for seven to ten minutes. If you need to, take a break.

5. Step down carefully and reassess your weight distribution and tightness.

Note: This exercise can be done without the slant board/wedge and is referred to as Wall Stand.

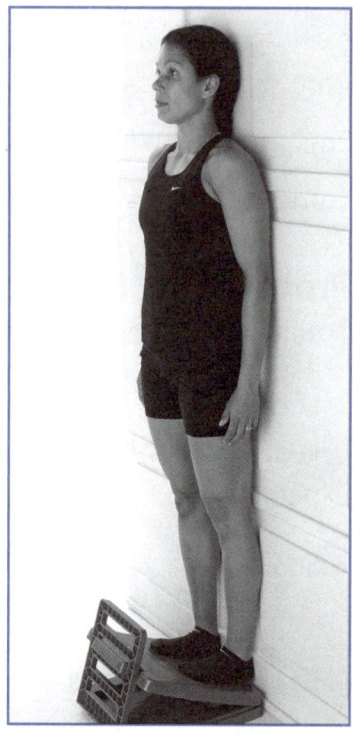
Wall Drop - Process 3

Treatment of Foot Symptoms

Muscle Cramps in Feet and Legs:
Muscle cramps can be caused by a variety of factors, including dehydration, calcium and/or potassium deficiency, and even engaging new patterns of movement during exercise. You might have experienced being awakened by a Charley Horse If this occurs, there are several remedies that may diminish the discomfort. While lying

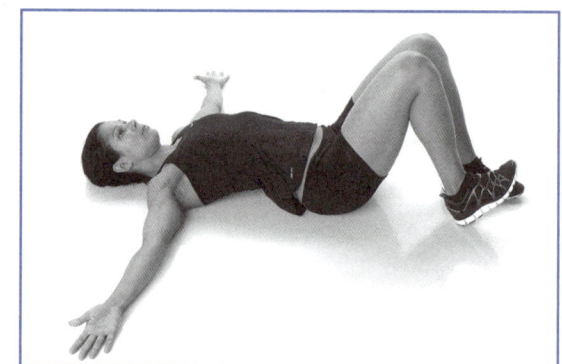
Muscle Cramps in Feet and Legs

Section 8: Foot/Ankle Processes

on your back, bend your knee, dorsi-flex your foot, and tilt your pelvis so you have an arch in your low back (anterior pelvic tilt). Hold this position until the cramp recedes. If you are standing and your foot or leg cramps, put pressure into the heel and directly up the long axis of the leg. Continue the pressure until the discomfort subsides.

Plantar Fasciitis:
Plantar fasciitis is defined as inflammation of the plantar fascia. There are multiple causes of plantar fasciitis including: bearing weight in the forward portion of the foot rather than the heels, pronated feet, and tight heel cords. To alleviate this problem, do one or more of the following exercises:

- **A. Wall Stand** Stand against a wall with your feet parallel and heels touching the wall. Allow your head and body to settle against the wall, and shift your weight into your heels for three to five minutes, building endurance if necessary.

- **B. Heel Cord Lengthening in Supine with Strap** (Section 8: Foot/Ankle Processes) page 77.

- **C. Gravity Drop** (Section 4: Multi-focal Processes) page 21.

- **D. Wall Drop** (Section 8: Foot/Ankle Processes) page 81.

- **E. Toe Raises Leaning on the Wall** (Section 8: Foot/Ankle Processes) page 81.

*Note: **Wall Drop**, **Wall Stand** and **Gravity Drop** are all essentially the same exercise but done on three different surfaces. They are all designed to redistribute weight toward the heels.*

Pronated feet:
To change the muscle imbalance associated with pronated feet:

- A. Do resistive ankle and foot exercise using therapy bands or straps in supination.

- B. Assume lunge position, making sure you are aligned from the foot to the top of the head. This helps produce medial-lateral stability from foot up. Other exercises that are helpful include:

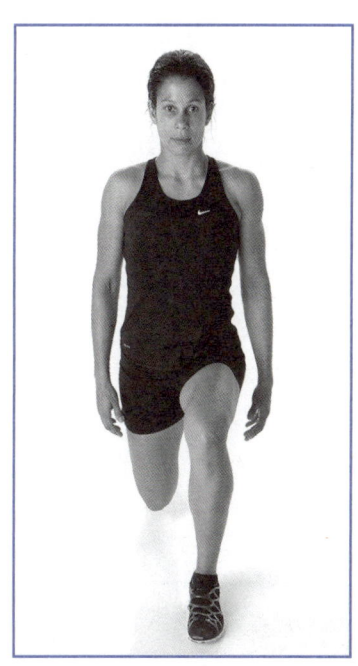

Pronated feet - B

C. Foot Circles (Section 8: Foot/Ankle Processes) page 75.

D. Inline Gluteals (Section 4: Multi-focal Processes) page 25.

E. Sit-to-stand (Section 4: Multi-focal Processes) page 28.

F. Sitting Floor (Section 4: Multi-focal Processes) page 29.

G. Static Back Pullbacks (Section 4: Multi-focal Processes) page 40.

H. Wall Sit (Section 4: Multi-focal Processes) page 50.

Shin Splints: Toes Raise Leaning on the Wall (Section 8: Foot/Ankle Processes) page 81.

Supinated feet: Dorsi- and Plantar Flexion with a Block in Sitting (Section 8: Foot/Ankle Processes) page 74. You can also do all the exercises listed above in Pronated Feet section as these exercises rebalance the feet into neutral.

My Progress Journal

Exercise Name	Date	Notes

Section 8: Foot/Ankle Processes

My Progress Journal		
Exercise Name	Date	Notes

Keep it up. Soon you will find a new normal!

Section 9: Knee Processes

■ Exercise – Pigeon-toed in Standing

Purpose: This process alters the muscular imbalance that is often associated with externally rotated hips, knees, and everted feet. The weakened muscles are stimulated in the pigeon-toed position, decreasing the demand on the external rotators.

Contraindications/Precautions: Consult your physician before doing this process if you have had recent knee or hip surgery.

Equipment: None

Process:

1. Assess the amount of discomfort in the knees. Rate the pain from one to ten with ten being the worst.

2. Stand upright with your feet in pigeon-toed position, hips aligned over your heels. Contract the quads at least fifteen to twenty times without engaging the gluteals or abdominals. Learning to activate your quads in isolation may take time. Keep practicing.

3. Reassess your knee pain. Do another set if necessary.

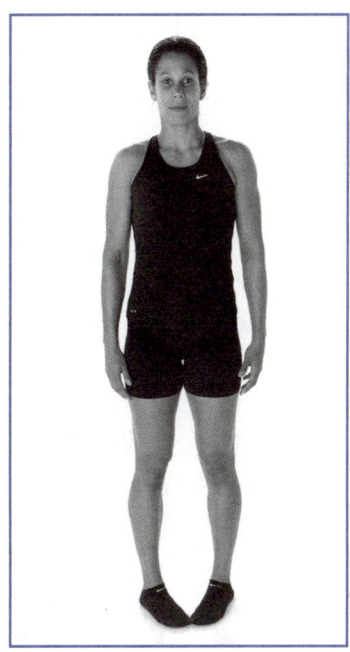

Pigeon-tied in Standing - Process 2

Power Over Pain Intelligent Fitness for the Amateur and Professional

■ Exercise – Side Lying Tensor Fascia Latae (TFL)/Iliotibial Tract (IT) Release with VersaStep

Purpose: The upper, outer thigh region contains a muscle called the tensor fascia latae that is in continuity with a ligamentous band called the Iliotibial tract. These two structures are crucial to the stability of the hip and knee. Many times this area becomes tightened and adhered to sacral, hip, femur, and outer knee structures. This exercise is designed to free adhesions and tightness of the TFL and IT.

Contraindications/Precautions: None

Equipment: VersaStep and a hand towel

Process:

1. Assess the degree of tightness and pain in the lateral knee and thigh along the femur upward to the outer hip. Rate the tightness from one to ten with ten being the worst.

2. Place a hand towel over the VersaStep. As you lie on your right side with your right leg straight, position the VersaStep at the upper, outer thigh. Flex your left leg at the hip and knee and place the left foot in front of the right leg.

3. Remain in this position for one to two minutes. Dorsi-flex the right foot then lift and lower the right leg by pushing the left foot into the floor.

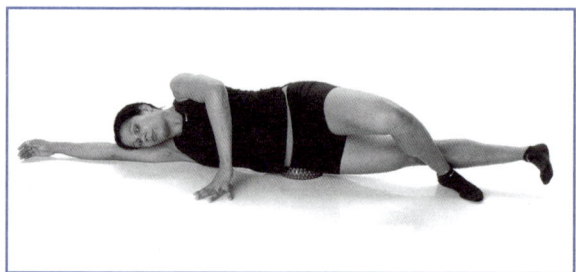

Side Lying Tensor Fascia Latae (TFL)/Iliotibial Tract (IT) Release with VersaStep - Process 3

4. If necessary, move the VersaStep downward toward the knee and continue the process of lifting and lowering the right leg.

5. Repeat this process lying on your left side.

6. Reassess the degree of tightness in the lateral thigh.

Section 9: Knee Processes

■ Exercise – Side Lying Unilateral Knee Extension
(Adapted from the Egoscue Method, 2001-2003)

Purpose: This exercise serves to activate the correct muscles of the hip and reposition and stabilize the knee. It also alleviates knee pain and discomfort, but you may have to complete several repetitions before pain is reduced.

Equipment: None

Contraindications/Precautions: If you have had recent knee surgery or knee replacement, consult your physician before doing this exercise.

Process:

1. Assess whether you have pain, discomfort, or dysfunction anywhere in the hips, knees, legs, ankles, or feet.

2. Lie on your right side with your right arm supporting your head, hips, and legs stacked one on top of the other, legs straight.

3. Keeping your right knee under the left, bend your right leg behind you to a ninety-degree angle. Turn your left foot so that your toes point downward and your heel is directed upward.

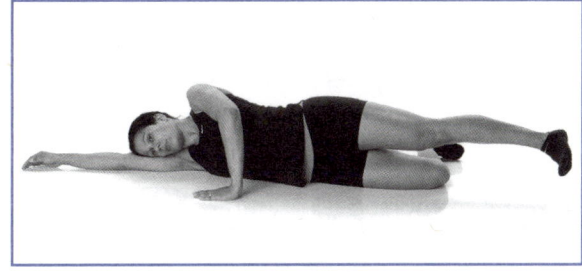

Side Lying Unilateral Knee Extension - Process 3

4. Bend the left knee, moving your foot towards your left buttock. Then return your left leg to full knee extension, remembering to keep your toes downward and heel upward. Continue to move your left leg in this manner for one to two minutes.

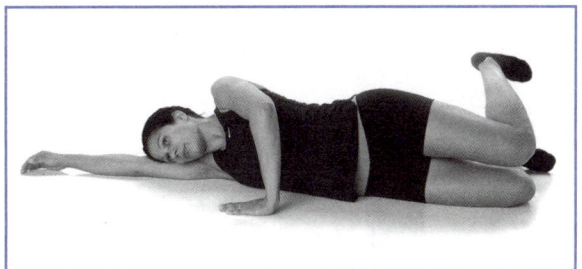

Side Lying Unilateral Knee Extension - Process 4

5. Repeat #2 #4 while lying on your left side.

6. Reassess your pain, discomfort, and dysfunction anywhere in the hips, knees, legs, ankles, or feet.

■ Exercise – Sitting Floor with Leg Lifts
(Adapted from the Egoscue Method, 2001-2003)

Purpose: This exercise is designed to modify the muscular imbalance that often creates an outward rotating knee and foot. This realignment reduces the torque on the knee and therefore reduces discomfort.

Contraindications/Precautions: If you have sciatic pain, this process may exacerbate the problem. If you have disc dysfunction, the process may make it worse. However, if your sacroiliac joint is out of alignment and causing sciatic symptoms, Sitting Floor may help you feel better.

Process:

1. Assess the amount of discomfort you have in the lower extremities, particularly in the knees. Rate the pain from one to ten with ten being the worst.

2. Find a flat surfaced wall or door. Sit and position yourself so that the back of your hips are as close to the wall as possible, legs stretched out in full knee extension and toes pointed toward the ceiling. Head is centered over the shoulders and shoulder blades are pressed into the wall. Palms up on your thighs. This is called long sitting.

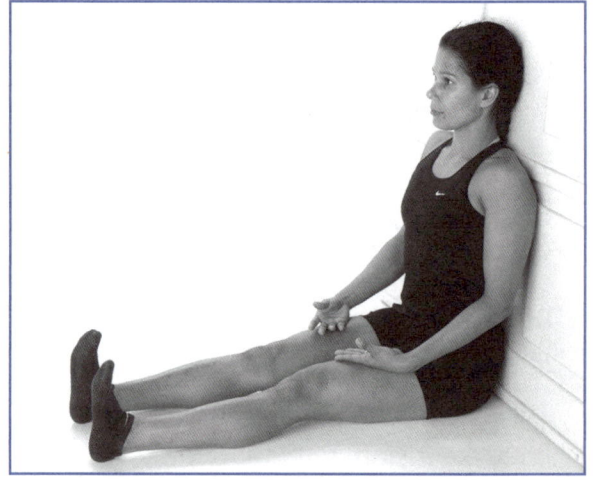
Sitting Floor with Leg Lifts - Process 2

3. Maintain this position for two minutes. If your hamstrings are extremely tight, do quad contractions.

4. Keeping the left leg still, lift the right leg off the floor then immediately lower it without leaning or pushing with your hands. Ideally, repeat lifting and lowering the right leg twelve to fifteen times.

Section 9: Knee Processes

5. Keeping the right leg still, repeat the process with the left leg.

6. Reassess the discomfort in your lower extremities with emphasis on the knees.

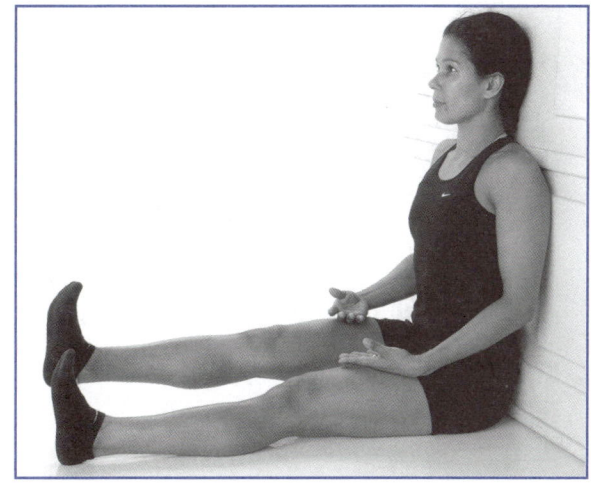
Sitting Floor with Leg Lifts - Process 4

■ Exercise – Soft Tissue Knee Balance

Purpose: This process is designed to balance the soft tissues around the knee joint. It also reduces knee stiffness and discomfort.

Equipment: A hand towel rolled lengthwise

Contraindications: None

Process:

1. Assess the degree of knee stiffness and/or discomfort. Rate it from one to ten with ten being the worst.

2. Sit on the floor with both legs extended. Slide a towel under the left knee, just above the crease. The towel itself provides a gentle upward pressure.

3. Place both hands on the tibia, the bone right below the kneecap, and apply gentle downward pressure. Hold for ten seconds.

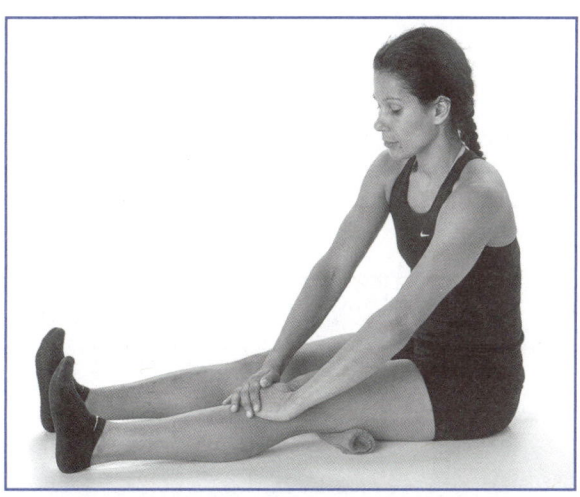
Soft Tissue Knee Balance - Process 3

Power Over Pain Intelligent Fitness for the Amateur and Professional

4. Slide the towel below the knee crease, place your hands above the knee on the lower end of the thigh, and apply gentle downward pressure. Hold for ten seconds.

5. Assess the degree of stiffness and/or discomfort in your left knee, and if necessary, use the towel and pressure to reduce stiffness and discomfort as outlined above.

6. Reassess knee stiffness. If necessary, repeat the process.

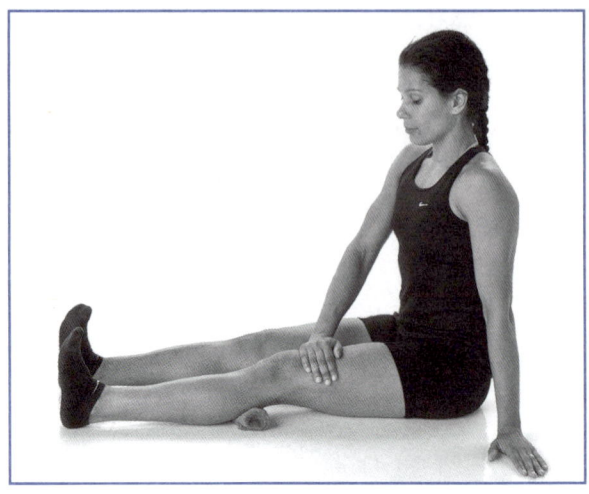

Soft Tissue Knee Balance - Process 4

My Progress Journal

Exercise Name	Date	Notes

Section 9: Knee Processes

My Progress Journal		
Exercise Name	**Date**	**Notes**

You have taken the first step. Don't stop now!

Section 10: Hip/Low Back Stability Processes

■ Exercise - Asymmetrical Horizontal Roll

Purpose of this exercise: This exercise is designed to address pain in any of the following areas: ankles, feet, knees, pelvic floor, hips, sacroiliac (SI) joint, back, and shoulders.

Equipment: VersaStep, massage ball

Contraindications: None

Process:

1. Start by rating your hip pain from one to ten with ten being the worst.

2. Lie supine in bent knee position, arms out at shoulder level, palms up.

3. Insert a massage ball or VersaStep underneath the right SI joint and extend the right leg, making sure that the right foot stays in line with the right hip. The left knee and foot remain in bent knee position.

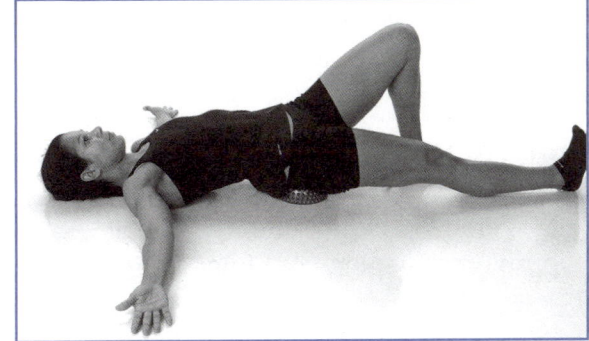

Asymmetrical Horizontal Roll - Process 3

4. Begin by pushing through the left heel and slowly rolling the right hip to the right. Continue the line of pressure up through the trunk to the right shoulder. Return pressure wave back down to the right hip, and then roll horizontally onto the left hip. Repeat this movement several times until you feel the change, at least two to three minutes.

Power Over Pain Intelligent Fitness for the Amateur and Professional

5. Move equipment to the left SI joint and repeat the same process with the left leg extended.

6. Slide the ball or VersaStep out from under your hips and reassess your hip pain.

Note: This exercise is effective for those with tightness and discomfort in the piriformis muscle.

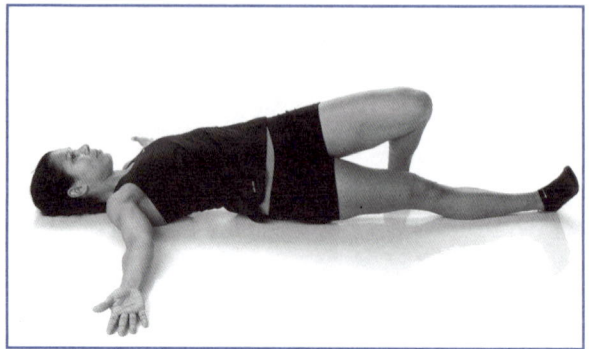

Asymmetrical Horizontal Roll - Process 4

■ Exercise – Bilateral Horizontal Roll

Purpose: This exercise is designed to address pain in any of the following areas: ankles, feet, knees, pelvic floor, hips, sacroiliac (SI) joint, back, and shoulders.

Equipment: VersaStep, massage ball, FitPAWS Paw Pods, yoga block

Contraindications/Precautions: None

Process:

1. Start by rating your hip pain from one to ten with ten being the worst.

2. Lie supine bent knee position. Insert a yoga block between your knees if you have problems keeping your knees together.

3. Insert a massage ball or a VersaStep centered above the gluteals and tailbone on the body midline.

4. Drop your knees together to the left, slowly rolling the left hip over the ball, then drop knees to the right, rolling the right hip over the ball. You may place a yoga block or pillow between your knees to keep them together.

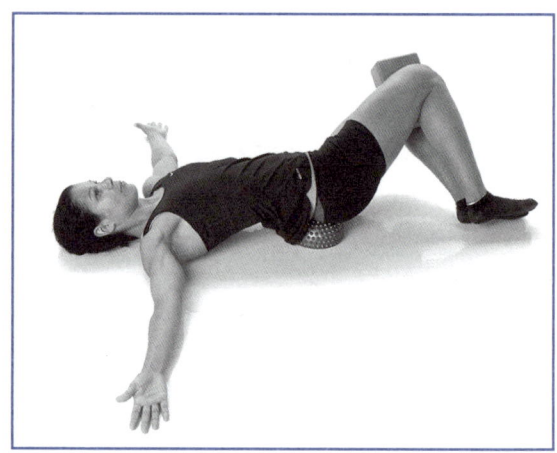

Bilateral Horizontal Roll - Process 4

Section 10: Hip/Low Back Stability Processes

5. Repeat this movement in both directions several times.

6. Slide the ball out from under your hips and reassess your hip pain.

Note: This exercise can be done with two VersaSteps, placing them side by side on either side of the midline above the gluteals and tailbone.

■ Exercise - Bilateral Horizontal Roll in Frog

Purpose: This exercise is designed to address pain in any of the following areas: ankles, feet, knees, pelvic floor, hips, sacroiliac (SI) joint, back, and shoulders.

Equipment: VersaStep, massage ball

Contraindications/Precautions: None

Process:

1. Lie supine with legs in frog and arms out to the side with palms up. Be mindful of any tightness in the hips, groin, low back, and shoulders. Start by rating your hip pain from one to ten with ten being the worst.

2. Place the VersaStep centered above the gluteals and tailbone on the body midline. The flat side of the VersaStep should be down. Reposition your legs in frog.

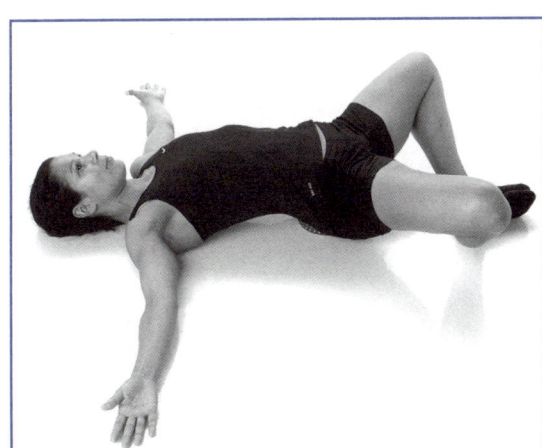

Bilateral Horizontal Roll in Frog - Process 2

3. Keeping the knees open, horizontally roll onto the right hip, return to midline, then roll onto the left hip, and return to the midline. Move slowly throughout the entire process. Repeat this movement series for two minutes or until hip or inner thigh tightness dissipates. Breathe evenly and deeply with each movement.

4. Remove the VersaStep and return to frog position.

5. Reassess pain and tight areas mentioned in #1.

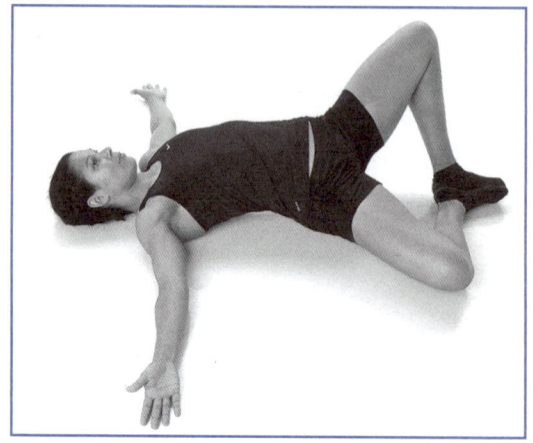
Bilateral Horizontal Roll in Frog - Process 3

■ Exercise – Bridging

Purpose: This process is designed for those with head/neck, shoulder, back, hip, knee, ankle, and foot pain. It provides bilateral reeducation for pelvic and core stability. It strengthens trunk and hip extensors and ultimately contributes to the synchrony used in gait.

Contraindications/Precautions: If you have low back pain, start by limiting your range of motion during bridging and check to make sure you are not rotating hips during the process. Once pain has dissipated, continue to increase the range of motion.

Process:

1. Start by assessing head/neck, shoulder, back, and/or hip pain from one to ten with ten being the worst.

2. Lie in supine bent knee position with the arms out to the side, palms open.

3. Keeping your feet flat on the floor, lift your hips as far as your body will allow, making sure the weight distribution is on your shoulders. Ideally, your shoulders, hips, and knees should align. Hold the position for three to five seconds. Take note of what you feel in

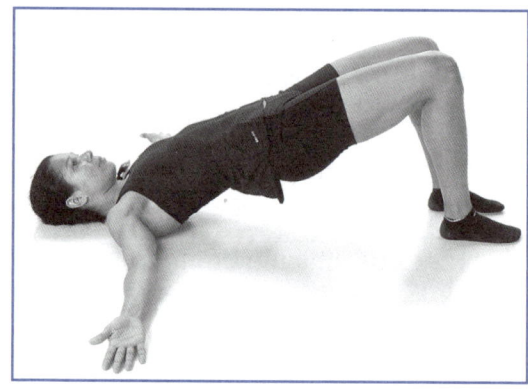
Bridging - Process 3

Section 10: Hip/Low Back Stability Processes

your knees, hips, back, shoulders, and neck. What changes do you note throughout the process?

4. Slowly lower your hips to the floor. Make sure you keep your hips level when lifting and lowering.

5. Continue to lift and lower the hips in a slow, controlled, steady rhythm.

6. Reassess your pain.

Modifications:

A. **Bridging with Yoga Block and Strap (Variation 1):** Assume the bridging position as in #2 above. Place a yoga block between your knees and a strap around your ankles. Keeping your feet flat on the floor, lift your hips as far as your body will allow while squeezing inward on the yoga block and pushing out against the ankle strap. Ideally, your shoulders, hips, and knees should align. Slowly lower your hips to the floor. Make sure you keep your hips level when lifting and lowering. Continue to lift and lower the hips in a slow controlled steady rhythm.

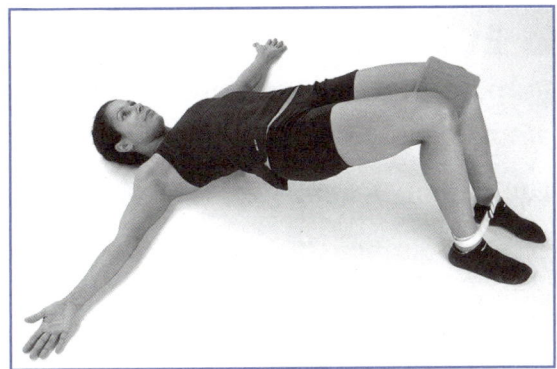
Bridging - Modification A

B. **Bridging with Yoga Block and Strap (Variation 2):** Assume the bridging position as in #2 above. Place a yoga block between your feet so that the long axis of the block is parallel to your feet. Place the strap around your lower thighs just above your knees so that your thighs are aligned with your feet. Keeping your feet flat on the floor, lift your hips as far as your body will allow while squeezing

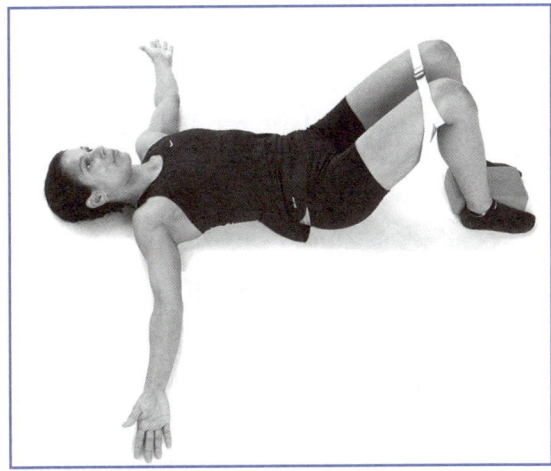
Bridging - Modification B

inward on the yoga block with your feet and pushing out against the strap with your thighs. Ideally, your shoulders, hips, and knees should align. Slowly lower your hips to the floor. Make sure you keep your hips level when lifting and lowering. Continue to lift and lower the hips in a slow controlled, steady rhythm.

C. **Bridging with VersaStep:** Lie in supine bent knee position with the arms out to the side, palms open. Place the VersaStep centered above the gluteals and tailbone on the body midline with the flat surface on the floor. If needed, cover the VersaStep with a small towel. Keeping your feet flat on the floor, lift your hips as far as your body will allow. Slowly lower your hips on to the VersaStep, allowing your hips to drop toward the floor. Make sure you keep your hips level when lifting and lowering them. Continue to lift and lower the hips in a slow controlled, steady rhythm.

■ Exercise- Hip Flexor Release with VersaStep

Purpose: This exercise is designed to reduce the tightness of the hip flexors and promote hip extension reciprocally.

Equipment: A VersaStep

Contraindications/Precautions: If you have had recent hip surgery, consult your physician.

Process:

1. Assess the tightness of your hip flexors by standing with your feet under your hips and palpate your groin. Note if the groin region is hard and/or indented at the hip/leg crease, indicating increased hip flexor tightness. Rate the amount of tightness from one to ten with ten being the tightest.

2. Lie face down and place the VersaStep textured side up into your right groin. Make sure your right leg and foot are lined up with your right hip. Place your forehead on your hands and bend your left leg out to the left side in a half frog position. Breathe and allow your

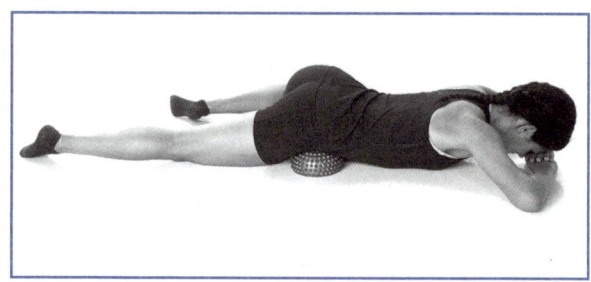

Hip Flexor Release with VersaStep - Process 2

Section 10: Hip/Low Back Stability Processes

right hip to settle into the VersaStep for one minute.

3. Slowly roll your hips from right to left at least one to two minutes. Then push your right foot into the floor, moving your body in upward and downward directions, further releasing the hip flexors.

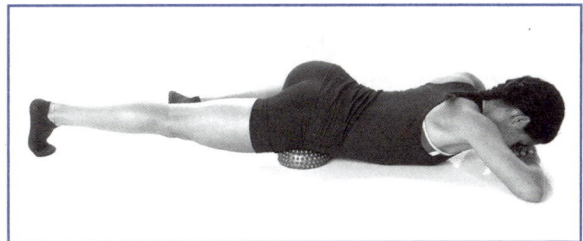

Hip Flexor Release with VersaStep - Process 3

4. Reassess your hip flexor tightness as in #1.

■ Exercise – Medial and Lateral Hip Stabilization

Purpose: This process helps to stabilize and reeducate the muscles of the hips and low back.

Equipment: A yoga block and a yoga strap

Contraindications/Precautions: None

Process:

1. Can you walk on a treadmill without holding on? If not, you probably have a degree of hip instability. Have someone videotape you walking away from and toward the video camera. View the video and note the quality of your leg swing. Are your feet straight ahead as you step and as your leg swings? Do your knees stay in line with your hip joints? Does your torso stay vertical over your hips?

2. Sit on the floor, bend your knees, and place a yoga strap above them. Tighten it so that your knees are in line with your hip joints. Then place a yoga block between your feet as illustrated in the photo. Now lie in supine, arms away from your sides with palms up.

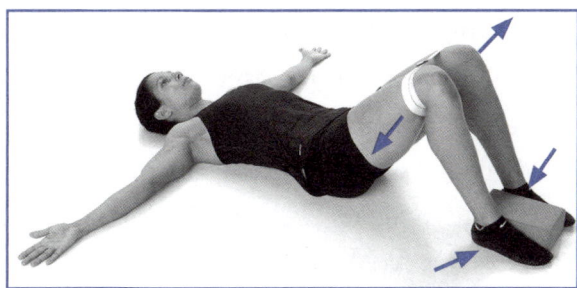

Medial and Lateral Hip Stabilization - Process 2

Power Over Pain Intelligent Fitness for the Amateur and Professional

3. Without using your abdominal muscles, simultaneously pull out against the strap at your knees and squeeze the yoga block with your feet. Keep your feet flat on the floor and your torso relaxed. Hold for two to three seconds and then release. Repeat this action at least twenty-five to thirty times. Note the amount of movement you have in the hips and legs while doing this exercise, indicating hip instability. This movement should decrease with increased repetition.

4. Reassess, noting whether your hip stability has changed compared to your initial assessment.

Modification:

Medial and Lateral Hip Stabilization with Reverse Located Equipment: Move the strap from above your knees to around your ankles, so that your feet and ankles are hip joint distance apart. Place the yoga block between your knees as depicted in the photograph. Keeping your feet flat on the floor, simultaneously squeeze the block and pull out against the yoga strap. Release then repeat the motion twenty-five to thirty times.

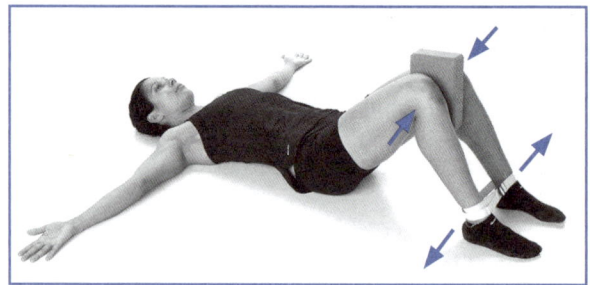

Medial and Lateral Hip Stabilization - Modification

Note: Both the exercise and modification above can be done by lifting and lowering the feet a few inches from the ground instead of keeping the feet stationary. This movement correctly engages the hip flexors. It is recommended that you do the stabilization exercise without lifting the feet before engaging your hip flexors. If your low back comes off the floor when you lift your feet, engage your low abdominals before lifting.

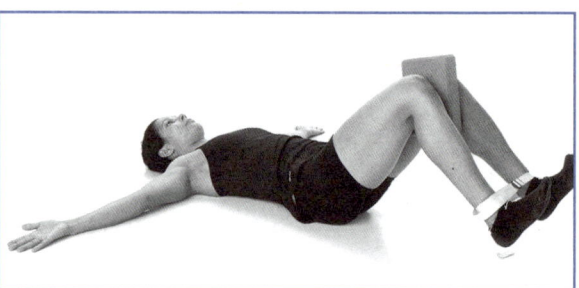

Medial and Lateral Hip Stabilization - Modification Note

Section 10: Hip/Low Back Stability Processes

■ Exercise – Pelvic Tilts with VersaStep

Purpose: This is one of the primary exercises used for low back pain control, reducing hip rotation, and reeducation of the muscles of hips and low back.

Equipment: VersaStep, a small hand towel

Contraindications/Precautions: If you have been diagnosed with a herniated disc or have had lumbar fusion, proceed with caution. You may need a small towel to cover the textured side of the VersaStep if your lower back region is hypersensitive.

Process:

1. Rate the amount of pain and degree of tightness in your low back region from one to ten with ten being the worst.

2. Lie on your back with your knees bent and feet on the floor. Your feet should be parallel and heels in line with your sits bones. Place a VersaStep above the gluteals and tailbone on the body midline.

3. Allow your hips to settle on the VersaStep for one minute. Phase one: Tighten your lower abdominals and tilt your navel toward your chin. This is known as posterior pelvic tilt. This motion allows the low back to move closer to the floor as the lumbar muscles lengthen. Do not engage your gluteals during phase one.

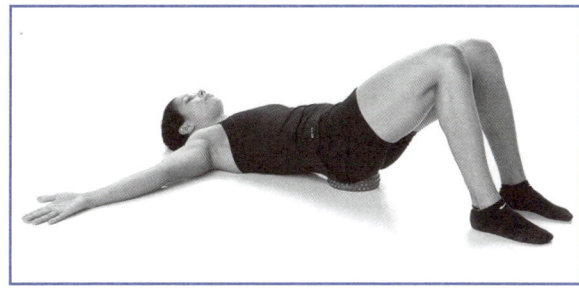

Pelvic Tilts with VersaStep - Process 3

4. Phase two: Shorten the muscles of the low back. This results in the low back lifting upward and the sit bones dropping toward the floor. This is known as anterior pelvic tilt.

5. Repeat phases one and two rhythmically and slowly, making sure to exhale during phase one and inhale during phase two. Continue these movements until you experience relief and decreased tightness in your back.

6. Reassess.

Modifications:

Pelvic Clock on the VersaStep: The Pelvic Clock on the VersaStep is an exercise adapted from Feldenkrais (Feldenkrais, 1972) Instead of just doing anterior and posterior pelvic tilts as described above, envision your hips lying on a large clock face. In phase one your hips tilt toward twelve o'clock. In phase two your hips tilt toward six o'clock. Slowly move between twelve and six o'clock ten to twelve times, and then progress to moving between one and seven o'clock, two and eight o'clock, three and nine o'clock, four and ten o'clock, and five and eleven o'clock. In each transition move your hips ten to twelve times on the VersaStep.

My Progress Journal

Exercise Name	Date	Notes

Section 10: Hip/Low Back Stability Processes

My Progress Journal		
Exercise Name	Date	Notes

How do you feel about your progress?

Section 11: Lower and Middle Thoracic Processes

■ Exercise – Counter Stretch

(Adapted from Egoscue Method, 2001-2003)

Purpose: This process serves to remove hip and trunk rotation and restore the normal spinal curve. It also helps to eliminate excessive hip flexion while discouraging maladaptive thoracic and shoulder patterns.

Equipment: A wall

Note: You can also use a counter or the back of a sturdy chair.

Contraindications/Precautions: If you have excessive limitation in range of motion of the upper trunk and shoulders, proceed with caution.

Process:

1. Assess the amount of tightness in your entire torso, shoulders, and hamstrings. Rate the tightness from one to ten with ten being the tightest.

2. Place your hands on a wall or table roughly shoulder height, and step back so that your arms are extended. Your feet should be parallel and directly under your hips with weight in your heels. Your hips are now approximately at ninety degrees of flexion. Drop your head and chest. The lower you place your hands on the wall, the more demand on the hips, torso, and shoulders.

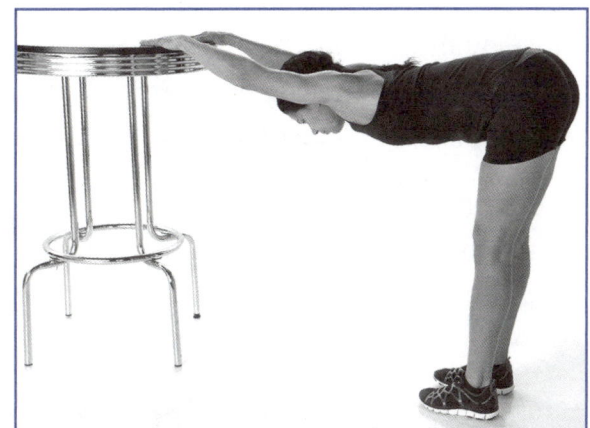

Counter Stretch - Process 2

3. For individuals who lack hip extension and have tight hamstrings, bend your knees slightly and concentrate on hip extension. Breathe and hold this position for up to one minute.

4. Stand up slowly and reassess your tightness.

■ Exercise – Crocodile
(adapted from Egoscue Method, 2001-2003)

Purpose: The purpose of this exercise is to promote voluntary bilateral rotation at the hip and spine while maintaining upper torso stability.

Equipment: None

Contraindications: If you have had hip replacement surgery, consult your physician.

Process:

1. Assess the tightness in your back and hips by lying in supine bent knees with arms extended to your sides at shoulder level, palms to the floor. Lift your knees and bring them over your hips. Keeping your knees and legs together, slowly lower them to the right, noting any tightness you feel in your lower torso and hips. Make sure you maintain your arms and shoulders flat to the floor during hip rotation. Return your bent legs to midline then repeat the assessment to your left side, noting tightness and/or limited range of motion.

2. Leaving your arms in the assessment position, extend both legs and place your right heel on top of the toes of your left foot.

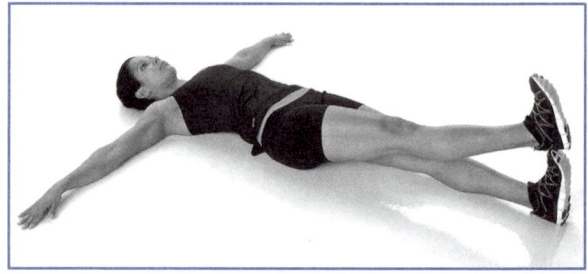

Crocodile - Process 2

3. Turn your head and look at your right hand. Keep your quads and hips tight and rotate your legs, hips, and lower torso to the left. Remember to keep your shoulders

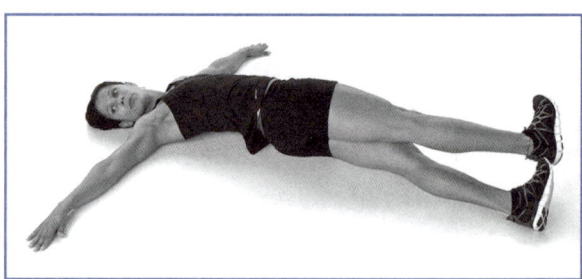

Crocodile - Process 3

Section 11: Lower and Middle Thoracic Processes

and arms flat to the floor. Stay in this position for at least one minute then return your legs and hips to center.

4. Now place your left heel on top of the toes of your right foot, turn your head and look at your left hand. Keep your quads and hips tight and rotate your legs, hips, and lower torso to the right. Hold this position for at least one minute.

5. Reassess the tightness in your back and hips as described in #1 above.

■ Exercise - Half Bridging

Purpose: This unilateral stretch helps to elongate the muscles of the torso and upper extremity while reducing flexion and tightness at the hip.

Equipment: None

Contraindications/Precautions: If you have had recent hip or shoulder surgery, consult your physician.

Process:

1. Assess the tightness and discomfort in your shoulders, hips and torso. Rate the amount from one to ten with ten being the tightest and worst discomfort.

2. Assume supine bent knee position in good alignment with your right arm at your side and your left arm fully extended above your head, palm up.

3. Push through your left heel, lift your left hip, and slide your left shoulder up toward your ear as far as your body will allow. Hold this position for up to a minute. If holding this position is difficult, drop your left hip and relax your left shoulder for a few seconds then resume the hip lift and shoulder reach.

4. Repeat this process on the right side of your body.

5. Reassess your tightness and discomfort.

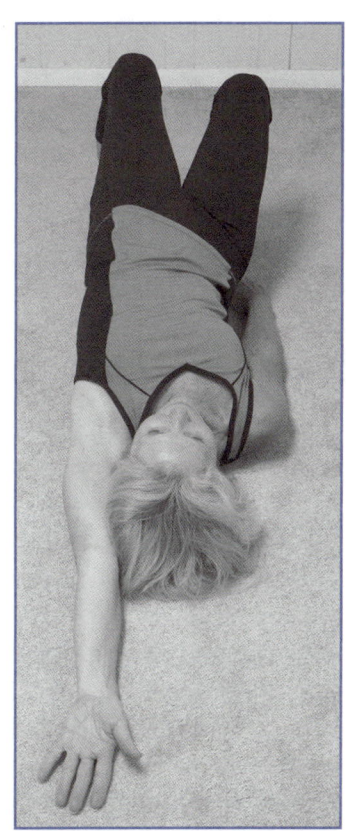

Half Bridging - Process 3

Power Over Pain Intelligent Fitness for the Amateur and Professional

■ Exercise – Prone Body Gliding:

Purpose: This process lengthens the muscles of the hips, torso, and shoulders, reducing tightness and discomfort.

Equipment: None

Contraindications/Precautions: If you have had recent shoulder surgery or have excessive tightness in the shoulder girdle, proceed with caution.

Process:

1. Assess the tightness and discomfort in your shoulders, hips, and torso. Rate the amount from one to ten with ten being the tightest and worst discomfort.

2. Lie face down with your legs extended in line with your hips and your arms extended in front of you. Keeping all extremities on the floor, glide your right arm forward and your right hip and leg away from your torso. Hold that stretch for three to five seconds. Now glide your arm and leg on the left side and hold for three to five seconds. Continue gliding for eight to ten times on each side.

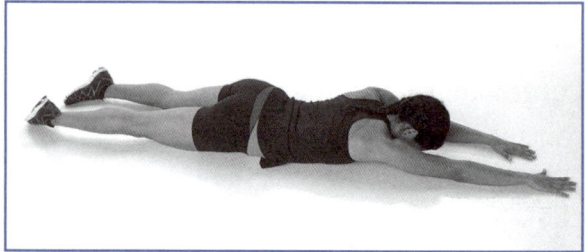
Prone Body Gliding - Process 2

3. Now glide your right arm and your left hip and leg, continuing to keep all extremities and your hips and torso in contact with the floor eight to ten times. Repeat this stretch with the left arm and right hip and leg eight to ten times.

4. Reassess your tightness and discomfort.

Section 11: Lower and Middle Thoracic Processes

■ Exercise – Prone Thoracic Muscular Reeducation:

Purpose: This exercise promotes reeducation of the muscles of the middle and upper back necessary for thoracic extension and proper postural alignment. It teaches you to lift your back, using your back muscles as primary movers instead of pushing with your arms.

Equipment: None

Contraindications/Precautions: None

Process:

1. Stand and have someone take a photo of you from the side. In side view, is the back of your ear lined up with your shoulder, hip, knee, and ankle joints? Is your upper back rounded? Is there tightness or discomfort between your shoulder blades? Rate your postural alignment, tightness. and discomfort from one to ten with ten being the worst alignment and the most uncomfortable.

2. Assume the prone position with your legs together, centered with your body midline. Bend your arms so that your forearms and palms are flat to the floor and your elbows are close to your torso. Your shoulders should be over your wrists if you are properly aligned.

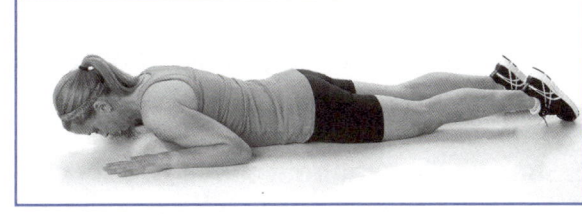

Prone Thoracic Muscular Reeducation - Process 2

3. Without pushing up with your forearms and hands, engage the muscles between your shoulder blades and lift your torso away from the floor. Hold this position for three to five seconds, keeping the shoulders down and away from your ears.

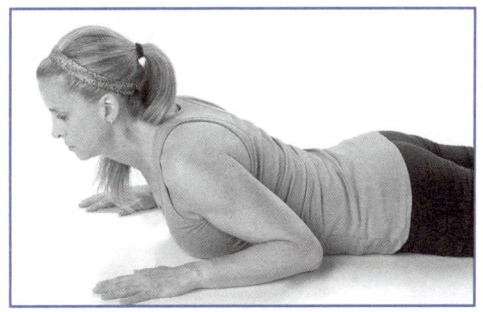

Prone Thoracic Muscular Reeducation - Process 3

4. Slowly lower your torso back to start position. Continue to lift and lower the torso as described in #3 for one to two minutes.

5. Stand and reassess your side view posture and the amount of tightness and discomfort. You might even have someone take an after picture for comparison.

■ Exercise – Sitting Thoracic Rotation:

Purpose: This process serves to encourage the scapula to glide back toward the spine, a function that is vital for postural and shoulder stability. As the back muscles engage, the chest opens and stretches. This process improves the body's ability to voluntarily rotate at the torso and promotes hip stability.

Equipment: A stable chair with a back, yoga block

Contraindications/Precautions: None so long as you listen to your body and do not force rotation.

Process:

1. Assess your ability to rotate your torso by sitting on the edge of a chair with your feet parallel, four to six inches apart and firmly planted. Sitting upright, align your head and torso over your hips. Rotate your head and torso to the right as far as your can; are you able to look over your right shoulder? Rate the ease of rotation from one to ten with ten being the hardest to achieve. Return to the front and repeat this process on your left side, rating left-sided rotation from one to ten with ten being the hardest to achieve.

2. Straddle the right front corner of your chair and place a yoga block between your knees. Your feet should be parallel and under your knees. Rotate your trunk to the right and reach for the back of the chair placing your hands on either side of the chair back. Hold this position for thirty to sixty seconds. Do not force the rotation beyond your body's capability. Repeat rotation to the right three to four times before returning to the front of the chair.

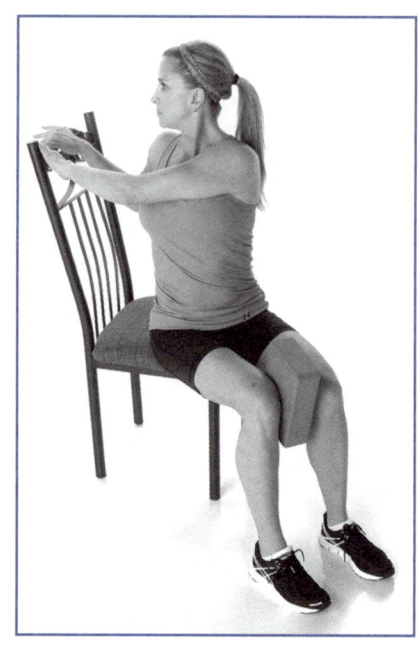

Sitting Thoracic Rotation - Process 2

3. Repeat #2 straddling the left front corner of the seat and rotating to the left. Repeat rotation to the left three to four times before returning to the front of the chair.

4. Reassess.

Section 11: Lower and Middle Thoracic Processes

My Progress Journal		
Exercise Name	**Date**	**Notes**

Power Over Pain Intelligent Fitness for the Amateur and Professional

My Progress Journal

Exercise Name	Date	Notes

How are you sleeping these days?

Section 12: Upper Thoracic/Shoulder Processes

■ Exercise – Backwards Shoulder Rolls

Purpose: This exercise is designed to activate the muscles of the shoulder girdle, providing increased range of motion and stability.

Equipment: None necessary. You can hold lightweight dumbbells for added resistance.

Contraindications/Precautions: If you have had recent shoulder surgery, consult your physician.

Process:

1. Assess the tightness and range of motion around your shoulders. Rate each from one to ten with ten being the tightest and most limited range.

2. Sit toward the edge of your chair with your feet facing straight ahead and lined up under your knees. Your torso should be erect and centered over your hips, arms at your sides with your palms upright in your lap. Your head should be centered on your torso.

3. Gently and slowly circle your shoulders backward and downward repeatedly for one to two minutes.

Modification: This exercise can be done in standing with your arms at your sides, palms forward.

■ Exercise – Double Leg Drop with Mini-windmills

Purpose: This process serves to elongate and open a restricted ribcage by producing muscular equality in all planes of movement. Mini-windmills diminish a multitude of dysfunctional patterns throughout the body but specifically address the complex interaction between the shoulders, torso, diaphragm, and hips. This process has been given a five-star rating by our students.

Equipment: None except during modifications to the process

Contraindications/Precautions: Consult your physician if you have had recent shoulder or hip surgery.

Process:

1. Lie in supine with bent knees, hands behind your head, and elbows open. Assess your ability to lower your shoulder blades and elbows to the floor.

2. Place your right heel on top of the left knee and drop both legs to the left as far as your body will allow. Maintain your torso and arm position as in #1.

3. Keeping your head in neutral, slowly slide your left elbow toward your left hip as far as you can, and then return to center. Then slide your right elbow toward your right hip and return to center. Note whether it is easier to move one direction over the other. Repeat for at least one to two minutes, depending on the amount of tightness and restriction. Return to supine with bent knee position.

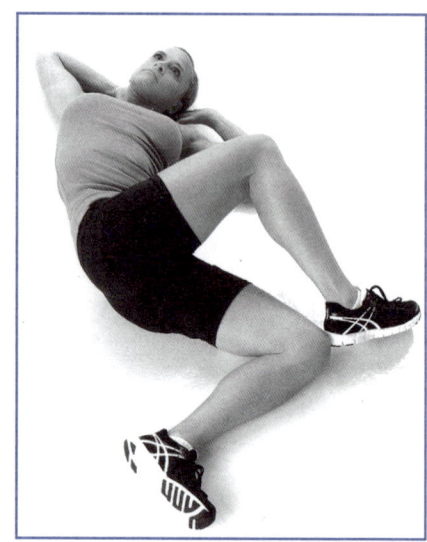

Double Leg Drop with Mini-windmills - Process 2

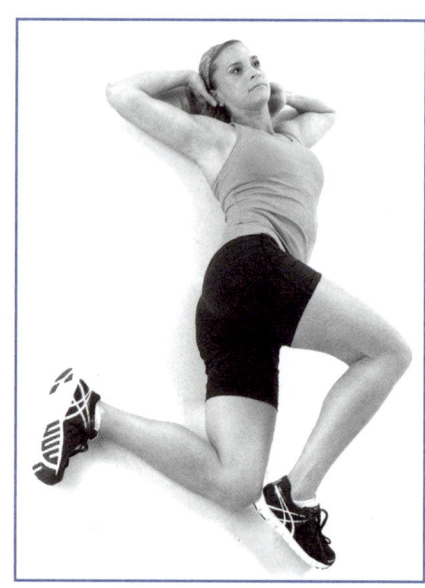

Double Leg Drop with Mini-windmills - Process 3

Section 12: Upper Thoracic/Shoulder Processes

4. Place your left heel on top of your right knee and drop both legs to the right as far as your body will allow. Maintain your torso and arm position as in #1.

5. Keeping your head in neutral, slowly slide your left elbow toward your left hip as far as you can and then return to center. Then slide your right elbow toward your right hip and return to center. Repeat for at least one to two minutes, depending on the amount of tightness and restriction. Return to supine with bent knee position.

6. Steps #2 to #5 constitute one full cycle. Repeat at least one more full cycle.

7. Reassess and note whether your ability to lower your shoulder blades and elbows has improved.

Modification:

A. Mini-windmills in Supine Bent Knees: If the Double Leg Drop position is too difficult for you, return to supine with bent knees position and do the Mini-windmill cycles without lower extremity involvement.

B. Frog with Mini-windmills: Start the process by sitting on the floor, placing the soles of your feet together. Make sure your feet are centered with your pelvis. Lie back allowing your legs to drop open into Frog position. Place your hands behind your head with the elbows open. Follow the Mini-windmills instructions in steps #3 and #5 above.

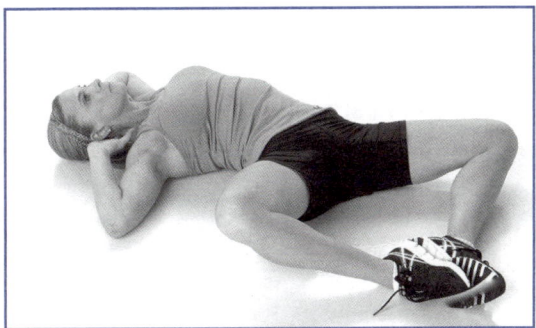

Double Leg Drop with Mini-windmills - Modification C

C. Frog Lateral Flexion with Mini-windmills: Follow instructions for modification B, adding lateral flexion so that the knee/hip moves up toward the shoulder/elbow, and the shoulder/elbow moves toward that same knee/hip, shortening that same body side.

■ Exercise – Shoulder And Arm Glide Progression

Purpose: This exercise is designed to stimulate all the muscles that move the shoulder blades and increase range of motion of the shoulder joint in the frontal/coronal anatomical plane of the body (Williams et al., 1989, p.13)

Equipment: Two VersaSteps, exercise tubing, small towel roll, and two hand towels to cover the textured side of the VersaStep.

Contraindications/Precautions: If you have chronic shoulder pain, do this exercise without using the VersaStep.

Process:

1. Lie in supine bent knee with arms bent at the elbow and tops of the forearms placed as close to the floor as possible. Assess the degree of tightness and your ability to lay your arms flat to the floor, using the one to ten scale with ten being the tightest and most difficult.

2. Remain in supine bent knee position and place a VersaStep textured side up under each shoulder. You may cover each of the VersaSteps with a towel if your skin is sensitive to the textured surface. The center of each VersaStep should be in line with the top of each scapula. Use a small pillow or towel roll under your head to keep your head and shoulders aligned. Place your arms palms up out to your side, and press the back of your shoulders into the VersaSteps. Repeat pressing into the VersaSteps twelve to fifteen times.

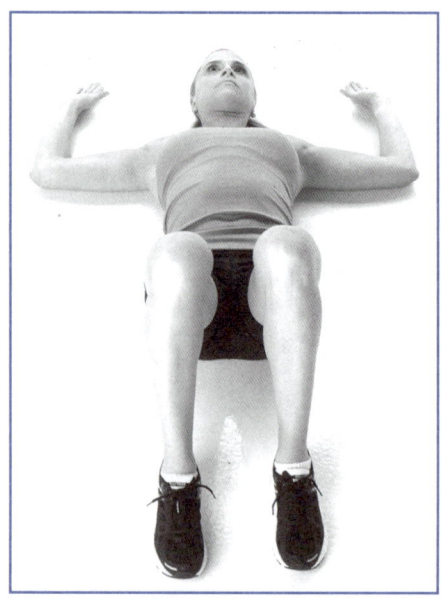

Shoulder And Arm Glide Progression - Process 1

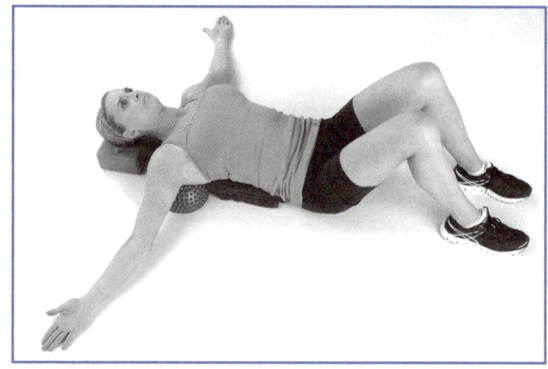

Shoulder And Arm Glide Progression - Process 2

Section 12: Upper Thoracic/Shoulder Processes

3. Now bend your arms at the elbow in an upright goalpost position. Press your elbows into the floor and elevate your sternum, making sure the back surfaces of your shoulders move closer to the floor. Repeat this action twelve to fifteen times. If this angle is too difficult, use the positions described in Walking Arm and Shoulder Presses later in this section.

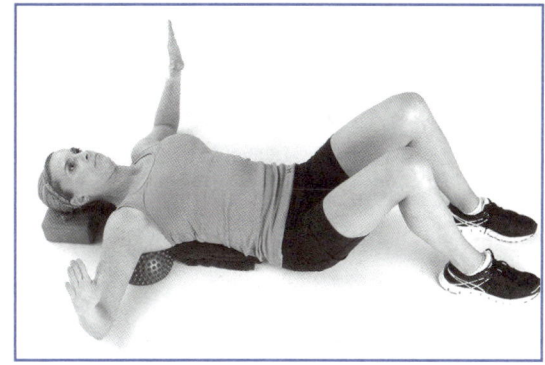

Shoulder And Arm Glide Progression - Process 3

4. Reposition your arms so that the tops of your forearms face the floor. Allow your arms and shoulders time to settle, noticing points that feel tight or strained. This is the start position. Slowly glide your arms towards your sides a few inches and return them to start position. Repeat arm gliding twelve to fifteen times.

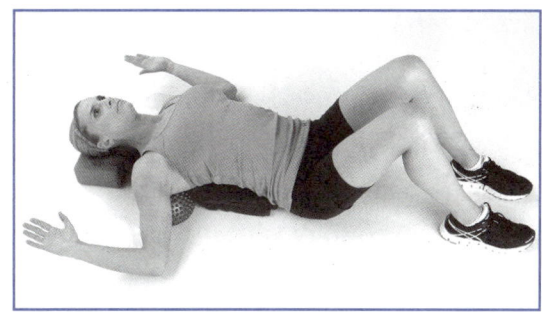

Shoulder And Arm Glide Progression - Process 3

5. If you are using the VersaSteps, remove them and reassess.

■ Exercise – Snow Angels

Purpose: This exercise increases range of motion and promotes the engagement of muscles of the shoulder girdle and upper extremities along with midline postural muscles of the upper thorax.

Equipment: None

Contraindications/Precautions: If you have chronic shoulder pain or have had recent shoulder surgery, begin with small range of motion and proceed with caution.

Process:

1. Assume supine bent knee position with arms out at shoulder level and palms up. Notice any tightness around the shoulder girdle and your weight distribution of your shoulders and arms in relationship to the floor. Also note what part of your shoulder blades and arms touches the floor. Rate your shoulder tightness from one to ten with ten being the tightest. Now rate the amount of contact your shoulders and shoulder blades have with the floor from one to ten with ten being the least contact.

2. Lie on your back in supine bent knee position with your arms out to your sides at a forty five-degree angle with palms up.

3. Engage the muscles between your shoulder blades and lift your sternum upward. Attempting to maintain contact with the floor, glide your arms bilaterally upward as far as you can and downward as if you were making Snow Angels. If you experience difficulty at any point in the range of motion, decrease your range of motion or slightly lift your arm off the floor and maintain the movement. Continue making Snow Angels with your arms for one to two minutes, working on increasing range of motion with each repetition.

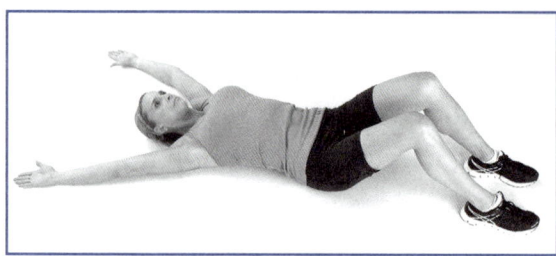

Snow Angels - Process 3

4. Reassess. Do your shoulders and shoulder blades make more contact with the floor? Has your shoulder tightness diminished?

Modification:

Snow Angels With Arms and Legs: You can open and close your legs as you move your arms. Note if your legs move bilaterally or if one of your legs moves more easily than the other.

Section 12: Upper Thoracic/Shoulder Processes

■ Exercise – Standing Thoracic Rotation with Extended Arm

Purpose: This exercise helps to dissipate thoracic pain and tightness around the shoulder blade and the outer side of the upper arm.

Equipment: A countertop or table, or any grounded surface at waist height, masking tape

Contraindications/Precautions: If your shoulder is unusually tight or painful, proceed slowly and with caution.

Process:

1. Stand with your left side about eighteen inches away from a countertop or table. Keeping your hips over your feet, bend at the waist with palm up, and extend your right arm as far as you can onto the countertop. As a reference point, you could place a piece of masking tape on the counter where the tips of your right fingers reached. Now repeat the process with your left arm, marking the location of the ends of the fingers on your left hand.

2. Stand with your right side next to the countertop, place your right forearm across your low back, and bend forward as you extend your left arm palm up, so that you can grasp the edge of the countertop. Drop your head and hold this position for one minute.

3. Repeat this process with your left side next to the countertop. Place your left forearm across your low back, and bend forward as you extend your right arm palm up so that you can grasp the edge of the countertop. Drop your head and hold this position for one minute.

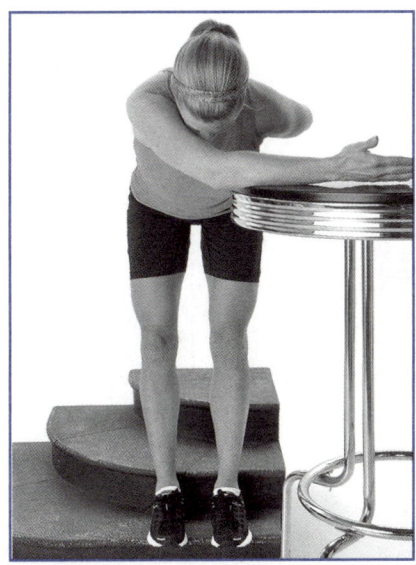

Standing Thoracic Rotation with Extended Arm - Process 1

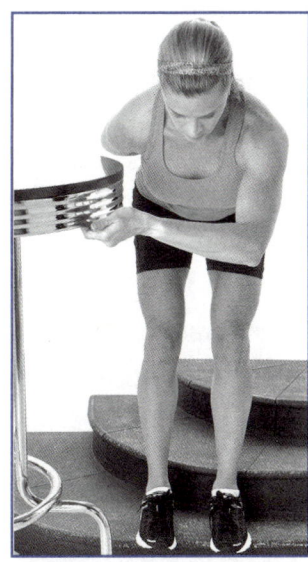

Standing Thoracic Rotation with Extended Arm - Process 2

4. Reassess, comparing the location of your fingertips on the countertop to the masking tape from the initial assessment for each arm.

■ Exercise – Sternum Tilts With Double VersaSteps

Purpose: This process enhances thoracic mobility and respiration.

Equipment: Two VersaSteps, a towel roll

Contraindications/Precautions: If you have spinal fusion, proceed with caution since this exercise promotes mobility in the torso.

Process:

1. Assess your ability to take a deep breath by inhaling through the nose and simultaneously timing the number of seconds you can inhale. Mentally note the time it took to inhale. Then while sitting in a chair, bend at the waist and lower your trunk and arms so that your chest touches your thighs as best you can. Hang your head and arms down toward the floor. Note the tightness you experience anywhere in the torso and rate that tightness from one to ten with ten being the tightest.

2. Place two VersaSteps on the floor, one above the other, approximately two inches apart. One VersaStep with textured side up should be placed above the gluteals and tailbone on the body midline. The textured side down VersaStep should be centered at the base of your ribcage. Arms to your sides, palms open. Breathe and allow the tightness in your hips and torso to subside.

3. Phase one: Tighten your low abdominals, and tilt your navel toward your chin known as posterior pelvic tilt. This motion allows the low back to move closer to the floor and promotes lengthening of tight midback and low back muscles. Do not engage your gluteals during phase one.

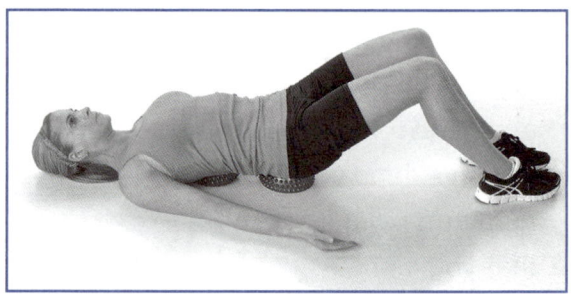

Sternum Tilts With Double VersaSteps - Process 3

4. Phase two: Shorten the muscles of the low back. This results in the low back lifting upward and the sits bones dropping toward the floor and is called anterior pelvic tilt. Be mindful of the increased mobility in your torso created by combining this movement with two VersaSteps.

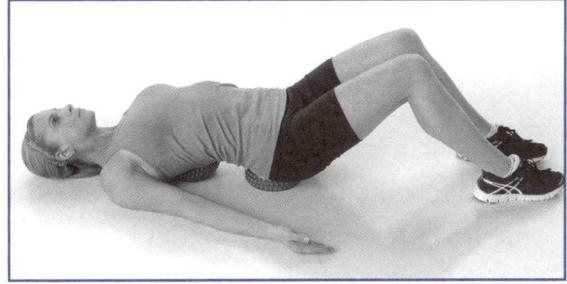

Sternum Tilts With Double VersaSteps - Process 4

5. Repeat phases one and two rhythmically and slowly, making sure to exhale during phase one and inhale during phase two. Continue these movements until you experience relief and decreased tightness in your back.

6. Reassess

■ Exercise – Upper Spinal Floor Twist
(Adapted from the Egoscue Method, 1998)

Purpose: This exercise enhances spinal rotation and the capability of the upper extremities and upper thorax to move into the same plane while the lower extremities and hips remain in neutral.

Equipment: None

Contraindications/Precautions: None

Process:

1. Assess your ability to turn your head and rotate your torso by sitting on the edge of a chair with your feet parallel, four to six inches apart, and firmly planted. Sitting upright, align your head and torso over your hips. Rotate your head and torso to the right as far as your can; are you able to look over your right shoulder? Rate the ease of rotation from one to ten with ten being the hardest to achieve. Return to the front and repeat this process on your left side, rating left-sided rotation from one to ten with ten being the hardest to achieve.

2. Lie on your right side with your knees and hips bent at ninety degree angles, legs and feet stacked on top of each other. Your arms should be on top of each other at shoulder level, perpendicular to your trunk.

Power Over Pain Intelligent Fitness for the Amateur and Professional

3. Bring your shoulder blades together and open your left arm to your left side, following your left arm with your head. Relax your left shoulder and allow the back of it to drop to the floor. Allow gravity to take over and hold this position for sixty to ninety seconds. If the intensity of the stretch is too much for the left shoulder, simply lower your left arm toward your feet or bend the left arm at the elbow and place your left hand just below your shoulder.

4. Repeat this process lying on your left side.

5. Reassess your ability to turn your head and rotate your torso as in #1.

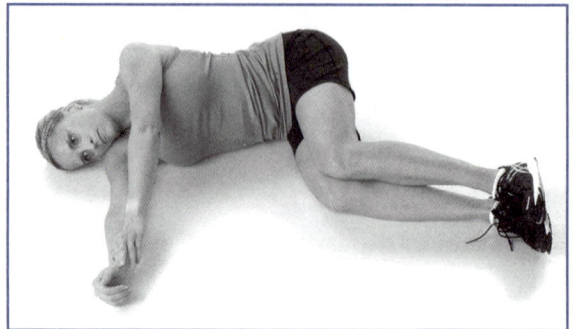
Upper Spinal Floor Twist - Process 2

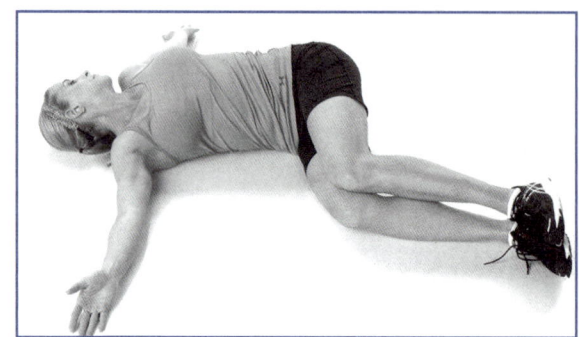

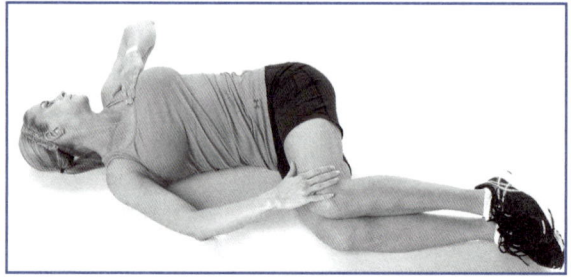
Upper Spinal Floor Twist - Process 3

■ Exercise – Walking Arm and Shoulder Presses

Purpose: This exercise progressively enhances bilateral shoulder retraction and shoulder stability from the midline outward.

Equipment: None

Contraindications/Precautions: None

Process:

1. Assume supine bent knee position with arms out at shoulder level and palms up. Notice any tightness around the shoulder girdle and your weight distribution of

Section 12: Upper Thoracic/Shoulder Processes

your shoulders in relationship to the floor. Also note what part of your shoulder blades touches the floor. Rate your shoulder tightness from one to ten with ten being the tightest. Now rate the amount of contact your shoulders and shoulder blades have with the floor from one to ten with ten being the least contact.

2. Lie in supine bent knee position and bend your arms at the elbow in an upright goalpost position a few inches from your sides. Press your elbows into the floor and elevate your sternum, making sure the back surfaces of your shoulders move closer to the floor. Repeat this action ten to twelve times.

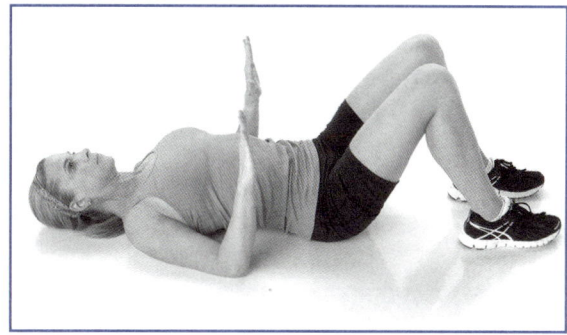

Walking Arm and Shoulder Presses - Process 2

3. Move your elbows a few inches more away from your sides and continue to press them into the floor ten to twelve times.

4. Now raise your arms so that they are perpendicular with your torso. Press your upper arms and elbows into the floor. Remember to elevate your sternum and let the backs of your shoulders drop closer to the floor. Repeat ten to twelve times.

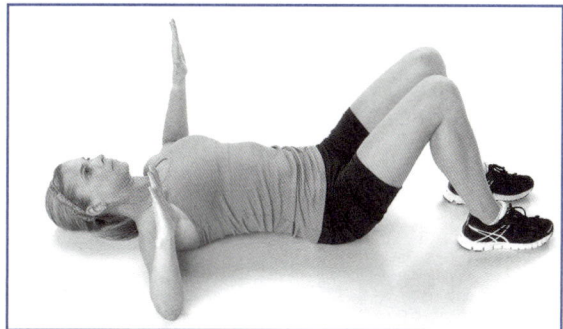

Walking Arm and Shoulder Presses - Process 4

5. Finally, elevate your arms and elbows one more time so that they are slightly above shoulder level. Continue to press into the floor ten to twelve times.

6. Reassess. Do your shoulders and shoulder blades make more contact with the floor? Has your shoulder tightness diminished?

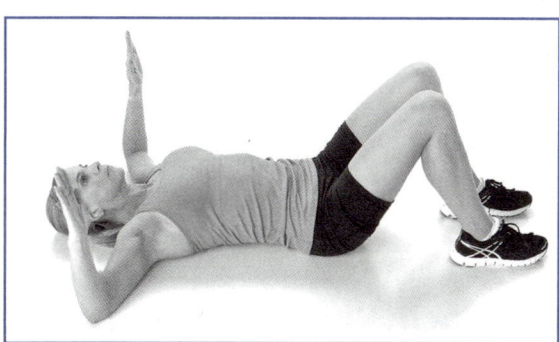

Walking Arm and Shoulder Presses - Process 5

Power Over Pain Intelligent Fitness for the Amateur and Professional

My Progress Journal

Exercise Name	Date	Notes

What activities are getting easier?

Section 13: Upper Extremity Processes

Introduction: By the time you reach this section of the manual, you have already engaged your upper extremities in numerous processes. This section provides you with additional material to further challenge your core muscles as you refine upper extremity skills.

■ Exercise – Back Stroking on the Stability Ball

Purpose: This exercise contributes to hip and low back stability, balance, and activates muscles of the core and shoulder girdle.

Equipment: Stability ball, one set of small dumbbells in the range of two to eight pounds. Check the Equipment Section of the manual to ensure that you have the proper size stability ball for your height, page 9.

Contraindications/Precautions: This is a more advanced balance and stability exercise and should not be done alone. We recommend that you attempt this exercise once you have successfully navigated the processes in the balance section of the book. If you have chronic shoulder problems, do not do this process while having acute pain. Establishing shoulder stability needs to come first.

Process:

1. Assess your ability to do this exercise by sitting on a stability ball and walking your feet forward while leaning back into the ball. Stop when your head, neck, shoulders, and upper torso are all in contact with the ball. The rest of your torso and legs will be self-supported. Your partner can check to ensure that your feet are parallel and even

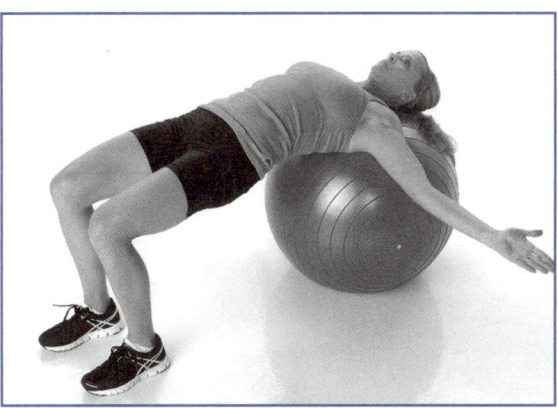

Back Stroking on the Stability Ball - Process 1

and your hips are level. Drop your left arm by your side and lift your right arm over your head. Switch your arms so that your right arm is by your side and your left arm is over your head. Rate the balance and stability of your torso on a scale of one to ten with ten being the least balanced or stable. Also rate the degree of difficulty placing and switching your arms from one to ten with ten being the most difficult.

2. Begin this exercise by returning to the assessment position. Have your partner make sure your feet are parallel and under your knees and your hips are level. Now have your partner hand you a set of dumbbells. It is better to start with lightweight dumbbells, allowing you to work a larger range of motion at the shoulder girdle.

3. Drop your left arm by your side and lift your right arm over your head. Switch your arms so that your right arm is by your side and your left arm is over your head. Concentrate on the muscles around and between your shoulder blades rather than on just moving your arms. Keep your arms straight but do no force range of motion.

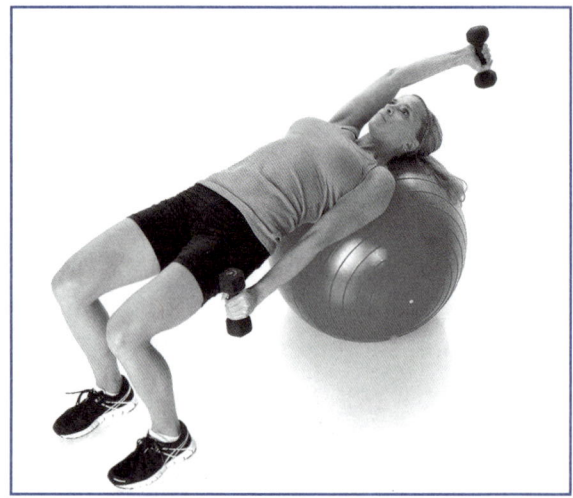

Back Stroking on the Stability Ball - Process 3

4. Repeat the arm pattern slowly, keeping your hip and torso level and still. Continue for one minute.

5. Reassess your balance and stability as well as the degree of difficulty placing and switching your arms.

Section 13: Upper Extremity Processes

■ Exercise – Unilateral Pullover with Resistance

Purpose: This exercise is designed to activate core musculature while unilaterally stabilizing the shoulder.

Equipment: A set of lightweight dumbbells two to six pounds, exercise tubing, light to medium resistance

Contraindications/Precautions: If you have chronic shoulder pain or recent shoulder surgery, use light resistance and proceed with caution.

Process:

1. Lie on your back and lift your arms over your head. Rate the degree of difficulty and tightness you experience in lifting your arms overhead. Use the one to ten scale for rating each arm/shoulder with ten being the most difficult and tightest.

2. Assume the supine bent knee position with your feet parallel and heels in line with your sits bones. Place a dumbbell in each hand, and extend your arms so that your hands are directly over your shoulder joints. This is called the start position. Engage the muscles between your shoulder blades and press your shoulder blades into the floor.

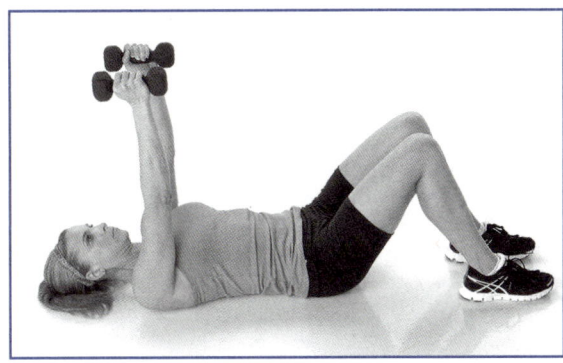

Unilateral Pullover with Resistance - Process 2

3. Keep the left arm stationary and slowly drop your right arm over your head as far as your body will allow, making sure your arm is straight and your shoulder blades maintain contact with the floor. Return your right arm to the start position. Repeat lowering and returning your right arm fifteen to twenty times. Be aware of your torso and hips, keeping them still while your arm is moving.

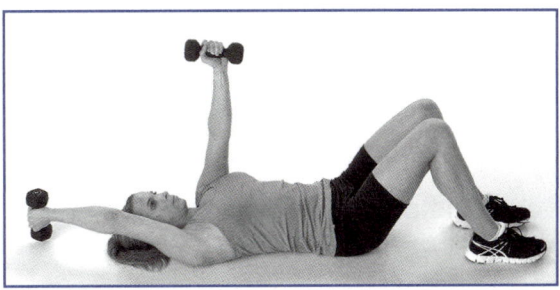

Unilateral Pullover with Resistance - Process 3

Power Over Pain Intelligent Fitness for the Amateur and Professional

4. Repeat this process with the right arm stationary and the left arm slowly moving. Repeat fifteen to twenty times.

5. Now lower your right arm to your side at shoulder level while slowly dropping your left arm overhead. Return your arms to start position as in #2 above. Now drop your left arm out to the side and your right arm overhead. Return your arms to start position. Be aware of any torso and hip movement that might occur as you move your arms in the various planes. Repeat these patterns at least fifteen to twenty times on each side.

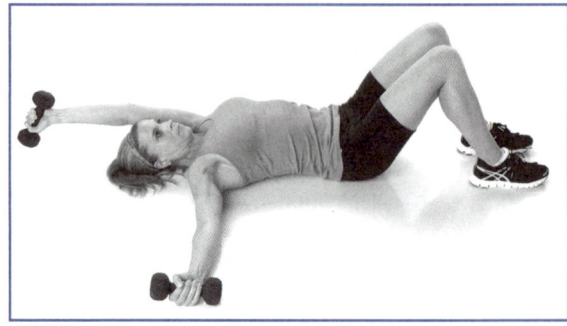

Unilateral Pullover with Resistance - Process 5

6. Reassess.

Modification: You can do this exercise while positioned on your knees on the floor or on a BOSU. You can also sit on a stability ball. Additional modifications include substituting resistance tubing for dumbbells and/or changing the plane of arm movement.

■ Exercise – Horizontal Unilateral Triceps

Purpose: This exercise is effective in creating muscular balance biceps and the triceps while stabilizing the shoulder girdle. We have included this exercise because we see so many clients unable to straighten their arms due to imbalance among the muscles of the chest, upper extremities, upper back, and shoulders.

Equipment: Exercise tubing, light to heavy resistance

Contraindications/Precautions: None

Section 13: Upper Extremity Processes

Process:

1. Lie in supine bent knee position and place your arms in upright goalpost position. Now lower your forearms to the floor, noting the degree of difficulty you experience in lowering your arms as well as the pattern of tightness down your arm. Rate the degree of difficulty extending your arms from one to ten with ten being the most difficult and tightest. What areas of the shoulder, arm, wrist, and hand make contact with the floor?

2. While in supine bent knee position, hold the handle of the exercise tubing in your right hand with your fingers facing the body midline, and grasp the tube with your left hand approximately twenty-four inches from the handle. This is known as start position.

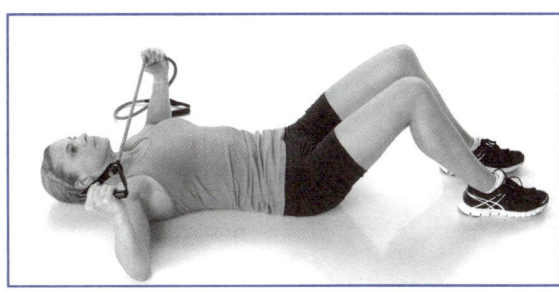
Horizontal Unilateral Triceps - Process 2

3. Stabilize both shoulder blades by pressing them into the floor. Using your right triceps rather than your right hand, lower the back of your right forearm to the floor with the palm open and your thumb hooked around the handle. Return to start position. Repeat this action fifteen to twenty times, continuing to stabilize both shoulders.

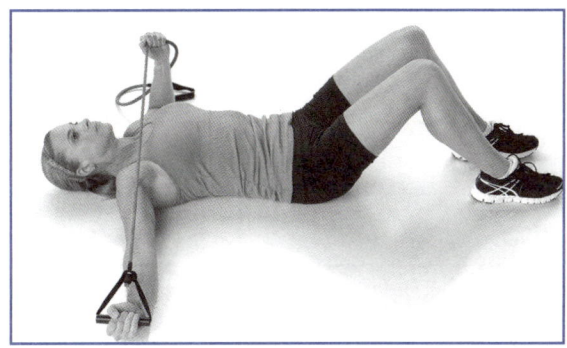
Horizontal Unilateral Triceps - Process 3

4. Now grasp the handle of the exercise tubing in your left hand and grab the tube with your right hand approximately twenty-four inches from the handle.

5. Using your left triceps rather than your left hand, lower the back of your left forearm to the floor with the palm open and your thumb hooked around the handle. Return to start position. Repeat this action fifteen to twenty times.

6. Reassess.

Power Over Pain Intelligent Fitness for the Amateur and Professional

My Progress Journal		
Exercise Name	**Date**	**Notes**

Resources are only valuable if you use them!

Section 14: Head/Neck Processes

Introduction: Many people of all ages have forward heads and pain in their cervical spines due to our technology-based culture. Hours and hours spent working at computer stations that have not been ergonomically customized contribute to widespread postural dysfunction. Therefore, we urge each of you to approach any head/neck exercise with care, monitoring your body's responses. Make sure you do not overstimulate this region. We recommend you start with fewer repetitions and assess the outcome before proceeding.

■ Exercise – Head/Neck Clock on VersaStep
(Feldenkrais, 1972)

Purpose: This exercise, adapted from Feldenkrais, is designed to balance the muscles around the neck and to increase range of motion of the cervical spine.

Equipment: A VersaStep and a small hand towel

Contraindications/Precautions: Monitor your body's responses frequently.

Process:

1. Sit on the front edge of a chair and look over your right shoulder. Note the quality of rotation you have when turning your head right. Now turn your head and look over your left shoulder, again noting the quality of rotation you have when turning left. Direct your gaze to the ceiling, allowing your head to drop back. Pay attention to any tightness or restriction. Drop your chin and look to the floor. Is there any tightness or discomfort during this movement? Rate each of the four head movements from one to ten with ten being the worst range of motion or most difficult movement.

Power Over Pain Intelligent Fitness for the Amateur and Professional

2. Cover the VersaStep with a small towel. Lie in supine bent knee and place the VersaStep at the base of your head at the cervical spine.

3. Envision that the back of your head is centered on a large clock face. Slowly move the top of your head up toward twelve o'clock then move your chin down toward six o'clock. Move between twelve and six o'clock ten to twelve times and then progress to moving between one and seven o'clock, two and eight o'clock, three and nine o'clock, four and ten o'clock, and five and eleven o'clock. In each transition, move your head ten to twelve times on the VersaStep, slowly inhaling and exhaling with each movement.

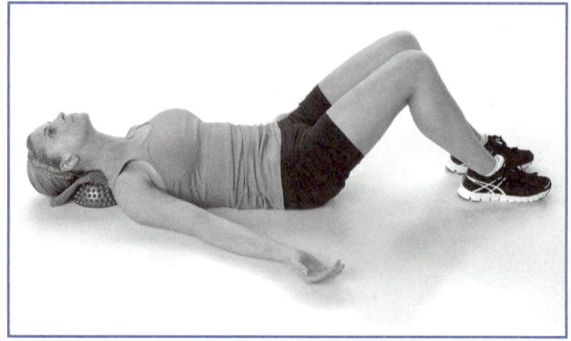
Head/Neck Clock on VersaStep - Process 2

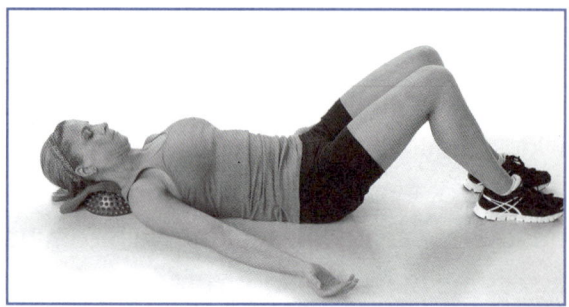
Head/Neck Clock on VersaStep - Process 3

4. Reassess the four movements described in #1 above.

■ Exercise – Static Extension Position
(Adapted from Egoscue Method, 2001-2003)

Purpose: This exercise is designed to increase thoracic and lumbar extension and aids in removing trunk and hip rotation.

Equipment: None

Contraindications/Precautions: If you have acute knee problems, consider padding your knees. For those with wrist restrictions, place your hands over three to four-inch-diameter firm balls. This will prevent the wrists from hyperextending.

Section 14: Head/Neck Processes

Process:

1. Assess the amount of pain or discomfort in the lumbosacral spine, under each of your scapula, and in your midback. Rate each area from one to ten with ten being the worst.

2. Start in the all-fours position and walk your hands forward about six inches. Shift your torso forward so that your shoulders are directly over your wrist and hands. Your hips should now be in front of your knees. Drop your head, pull your shoulder blades together, and extend your hips as best as you can.

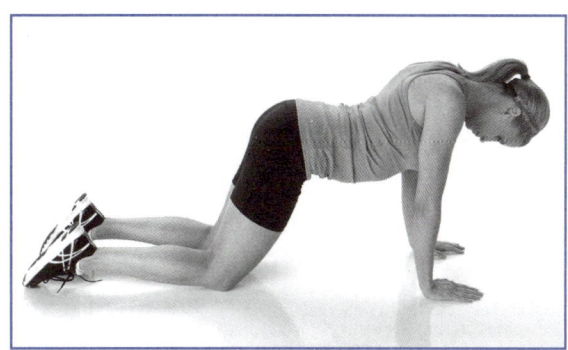

Static Extension Position - Process 2

3. Hold this position, working up to two minutes.

4. Reassess.

■ Exercise – Supine Feet-to-Head Release with VersaStep

Purpose: This process is designed to release tension in upper thoracic and cervical muscles. It also promotes muscular balance and removes inappropriate cervical rotation.

Equipment: A VersaStep and a small hand towel

Contraindications/Precautions: Monitor your body's responses frequently.

Process:

1. Sit on the front edge of a chair and look over your right shoulder. Note the quality of rotation you have when turning your head right. Now turn your head and look over your left shoulder, again noting the quality of rotation you have when turning left. Direct your gaze to the ceiling, allowing your head to drop back. Pay attention to any tightness or restriction. Drop your chin and look to the floor. Is there any tightness or discomfort during this movement? Rate each of the four head movements from one to ten with ten being the worst range of motion or most difficult movement.

2. Cover the VersaStep with a small towel. Lie in supine bent knee and center the VersaStep at the base of your head at the cervical spine. Place your arms at your sides with your palms up.

3. Push your weight through your heels upward toward the top of your head, allowing your head and neck to move gently and subtly over the VersaStep. Repeat the heel-to-head oscillation for two to three minutes or until your tightness has diminished.

4. Now press the back of your shoulders into the floor and slowly rotate your head to the left, keeping your neck from side bending and maintaining your chin away from your chest. Hold this position for sixty to ninety seconds and return your head to midline, making sure your head is centered.

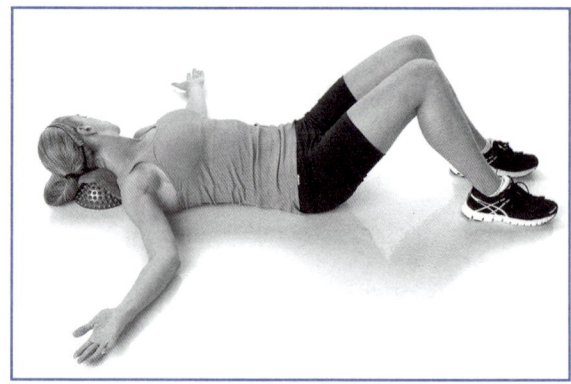

Supine Feet-to-Head Release with VersaStep - Process 4

5. Now rotate your head to the right, keeping your neck from side bending and maintaining your chin away from your chest. Hold this position for sixty to ninety seconds and return your head to midline, making sure your head is centered.

6. Repeat #4 and #5 again.

7. Reassess.

■ Exercise - Wall Towels
(Adapted from Egoscue Method, 1998)

Purpose: In this exercise, the towels serve to reeducate the cervical and lumbar spinal curves and provide sensory input. By standing with the towels against the wall, the ankles, knees, hips, and shoulders promote proper joint loading and thus help remove inappropriate trunk and hip rotation.

Equipment: Two bath towels each rolled into three to four-inch- diameter rollers.

Contraindications/Precautions: None

Section 14: Head/Neck Processes

Process:

1. Assess the discomfort and tightness in your neck, shoulders, torso, low back, hips, knees, ankles, and feet. Rate these areas from one to ten with ten being the worst.

2. Take the pre-rolled towels to a wall and stand with your back to the wall, inserting the towels perpendicular to the spine and behind the neck and lumbar region. Your heels need to be touching the wall and your feet should be parallel and hip joint distance apart. Your arms should be out to your sides, palms open.

3. Hold this position three to five minutes

4. Reassess your tightness and discomfort

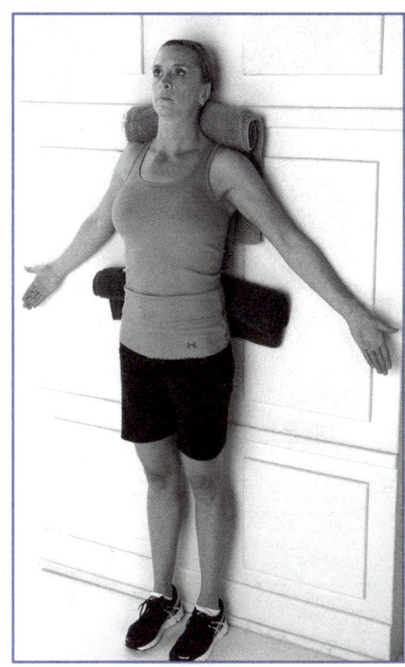

Wall Towels - Process 2

My Progress Journal		
Exercise Name	**Date**	**Notes**

Power Over Pain Intelligent Fitness for the Amateur and Professional

My Progress Journal		
Exercise Name	**Date**	**Notes**

Are you looking up more than you used to?

Section 15: Sequences of Exercises for Specific Areas of Function

Introduction: Each exercise in this manual has its own benefit; however, based on the specific problem being addressed, sometimes it is most advantageous to perform a group of exercises in a particular order. We have included a number of sequences below that have been effective for our clients.

Hip Sequence #1: This sequence is helpful to diminish rotation and reduce tightness in the low back, lower extremities and torso. **Static Wall,** page 41, **Static Wall Splits,** page 42, **Static Wall Flexion,** page 43 and **Frog,** page 19

Hip sequence #2: This sequence is designed to reeducate all load-bearing joints and promote improved bilateral function and increase flexion and extension of the spine. **Wall Sit,** page 50, **Inline Gluteals,** page 25, **Cats and Dogs,** page 16, **Prone Ankle Squeezes,** page 27 and **Triangle,** page 48

Shoulder Sequence #1: This sequence facilitates proper vertical loading and bilateral movement of the torso and upper extremities. It also supports coordination among the upper extremities, torso, and neck. **Walking Arm and Shoulder Presses,** page 124, **Frog Pullovers with a Strap,** page 21, **Standing Wall Clock,** page 34, and **Upper Spinal Floor Twist,** page 123

Shoulder Sequence #2: This sequence addresses tightness in the upper extremities and thorax while enhancing bilateral movement in the shoulders, upper, and middle back. **Walking Arm and Shoulder Presses,** page 124, **Sitting Floor Elbow Curls,** page 31, **Shoulder and Arm Glide Progression,** page 118, **Snow Angels,** page 119, **Upper Spinal Floor Twist,** page 123

Power Over Pain Intelligent Fitness for the Amateur and Professional

Scapular sequence: This sequence supports optimal movement and positioning of the scapula by engaging all of the muscles of the upper and midthorax.
Wall Presses, page 49, **Walking Arm and Shoulder Presses**, page 124, **Shoulder and Arm Glide Progression**, page 118, **Snow Angels**, page 119, **Back Stroking on the Stability Ball**, page 127

My Progress Journal		
Exercise Name	**Date**	**Notes**

Section 15: Sequences of Exercises for Specific Areas of Function

My Progress Journal		
Exercise Name	**Date**	**Notes**

Congratulations on your progress and remember you will continue to improve if you keep working!

Section 16: Bibliography/References

References:

Alon, R. (2010). *Bones For Life: Chairs Teacher's Manual*.
    Foundation For Movement Intelligence: Portland, ME.

Alon, R. (2007). *Bones For Life Teacher's Manual Segment I*.
    Foundation For Movement Intelligence: Portland, ME.

Alon, R. (2007). *Bones For Life Teacher's Manual Segment II*.
    Foundation For Movement Intelligence: Portland, ME.

Alon, R. (2007). *Bones For Life Teacher's Manual Segment III*.
    Foundation For Movement Intelligence: Portland, ME.

Alon, R. (2012). *Walk For Life Teacher's Manual I*.
    Foundation For Movement Intelligence: Portland, ME.

Egoscue, P. & Gittines, R. (1998). *Pain Free: A Revolutionary Method for Stopping Chronic Pain*. New York: Bantam.

Egoscue, P. & Gittines, R. (1999). *Pain Free at your PC*.
    New York: Bantam.

Egoscue, P. & Gittines, R (1992). *The Egoscue Method of Health Through Motion*.
    New York: HarperCollins.

Egoscue, P. (2001-2003). www.egoscue.com/WebMenus/ECiseHTML
    (Exercise Menu Available to Egoscue Specialists and Affiliates)

Feldenkrais, M. (1972). *Awareness Through Movement: Health Exercises for Personal Growth*.
   New York: Harper & Row.

Jenkins, D. (1991). *Hollinshead's Functional Anatomy of the Limbs and Back* (6th ed.)
   Philadelphia: W.B. Saunders Co.

Kendall, F., MCCreary, E., Provance, P., Rodgers, M., & Romani, W. (2005).
   Muscles Testing and Function With Posture and Pain (5th ed.).
   Baltimore: Lippincott Williams & Wilkins.

Overmyer, L. (2009). *Ortho-Bionomy A Path to Self Care*.
   Berkeley: North Atlantic Books.

Zemach-Bersin, D., Zemach-Bersin, K. & Reese, M. (1990).
   Relaxercise The Easy New Way To Health & Fitness.
   New York: HarperSanFrancisco – Division of HarperCollins.

Section 17: Glossary

Abduction: The anatomical term for moving a body part away from the body's midline.

Acute: Intense, sharp, stabbing pain; sudden onset.

Adaptive: The ability to make appropriate changes for the situation or condition required.

Adduction: The anatomical term for moving a body part toward the body's midline.

Agility: The capability to be nimble and active.

Alignment: The position of body parts in relationship to one another, as in postural alignment.

All Fours: quadruped.

Anterior: The front surface of the body.

Balance: To bring into equilibrium; the distribution of muscle around a joint.

Base of Support: The surface in contact with the ground on which the object balances.

Center of Gravity: The point at which the coronal, sagittal, and transverse planes all intersect; the point at which the mass of the body is equally distributed around it.

Chronic: Ongoing; constant; persisting over time.

Core: The center of a mass; most important part.

Coronal Plane: An anatomical term for the division of the body into a front section and a back section.

Dorsal: An anatomical term referring to the back surface of the body.

Dynamic Tension: Equal tension or pull between the front surface and back surface of the body.

Dysfunction: The inability to function any less than optimally.

Extension: An anatomical term that refers to activation of the muscles on the backside of the body; the straightening of a bent part.

Flexibility: The range of motion in a joint or series of joints; limber; mobile; supple; pliable.

Flexion: An anatomical term that refers to the activation of muscles on the front side of the body with the exception of the hamstring muscle, located on the back of the thighs that flexes the knee; the decrease of an angle between two parts.

Function: The characteristic activity of a specific joint, person, or thing.

Kinesthetic Sense: The ability to sense the weight distribution, movement, or position of a body part in space.

Kinetic Chain: Biomechanical connection between the joints in a movement sequence or pattern.

Kyphosis: An exaggerated rounding of the upper back, also known as round back or hunchback. It is usually associated with a forward head.

Lateral: Relating to, on, or toward the side.

Lateral Flexion: Side bending; lateral flexion can occur at multiple regions of the body including the head, torso, waist, and hips.

Load-bearing: Capability of a joint or series of joints to sustain gravity. The load-bearing joints must be aligned for optimal function.

Lordosis: Excessive inward curve of the lumbar spine, also known as swayback. The cervical spine, if excessively curved inward, may also be called lordotic. Both excessive inward curves are associated with a forward head.

Section 17: Glossary

Neutral: The point at which the tension is balanced on all sides of a joint or region without stress.

Maladaptive: Inappropriate response to the environment or to any stimulation.

Medial: Located inwards or extending toward the middle or midline.

Misalignment: Not optimally aligned; anything that deviates from the plumb line used to determine alignment.

Mobilize: To make mobile or capable of movement.

Posterior: Backside; opposite the front; same as dorsal.

Posterior Chain: A group of muscles, tendons, and ligaments located on the backside of the human body whose function is primarily hip and torso extension. Some of the main muscles in this group include: gluteals, hamstrings, erector spinae, gastrocnemius, external obliques, and multifidus.

Pronated Feet: An anatomical term referring to the inner arch and ankle of the foot collapsing toward the body midline. This condition can be congenital or acquired.

Prone: Lying face down.

Range of Motion: The ability of a joint to be moved passively or actively through its entire range. For example, the elbow is a hinge joint that moves between flexion and extension; therefore, its optimal range of motion would be from full flexion to full extension.

Rotation: Turning around a center or an axis.

Sacroiliac Joint: A joint in the bony pelvis on the posterior body side, formed by the sacrum and the ilium. This joint, also known as the SI joint, has strong ligaments that connect the sacrum to the ilium.

Sagittal Plane: Divides the body into a right side and a left side.

Sits Bones: The non-anatomical term for the ischial tuberosities, the lower back of the hipbones that bears the weight of the body in sitting.

Spasm: A sudden and involuntary contraction of a muscle that may also be associated with a sudden pain; a Charley Horse; cramp. Spasms result from a variety of causes and are usually temporary in nature.

Stabilize: To hold steady; firmly fixed and not easily altered.

Static: Fixed or stationary; not moving.

Strength: An attribute acquired by increasing the load over time; the ability to resist force or strain.

Supine: Lying on your back.

Supinated Feet: An anatomical term referring to misplaced weight distribution of the foot so that weight is on the outer borders of the feet and the long arches are higher than normal. This condition can be congenital or acquired.

Transverse Plane: Divides the body into a top half and a bottom half.

Trauma: Physical, emotional, or cognitive damage; wound caused by an extrinsic agent.

Ventral: The front surface of the body.

Notes

Notes